OPERATIVE SURGERY REVISION

OPERATIVE SURGERY REVISION

JOHN J. SHIPMAN,

M.B., L.R.C.P., M.S.(Lond.), F.R.C.S.(Eng.)

Senior Consultant Surgeon
The Lister Hospital, Stevenage
and
Associated Hospitals

THIRD EDITION

LONDON
H. K. LEWIS & CO. LTD.
1977

First published 1962
Second edition 1969
Third edition 1977

Standard Book No. 0 7186 0429 6

TO MY WIFE ELIZABETH

Printed in Great Britain by
The Whitefriars Press Ltd., London and Tonbridge

INTRODUCTION

The final part of Fellowship may be a stumbling block to the student and it is to help overcome this hurdle that this book on operative surgery has been compiled.

It is designed to be used in the revision of the essential steps carried out in a number of routine operations. This number has been kept to a minimum, but some rare operations are included which have occasionally been asked for in a Fellowship examination. An attempt has been made to condense the number of steps in each operation. Easily forgotten or important points are marked with an asterisk (*).

To use the book to the best advantage the student should first write down the steps of each operation and then check them against the text. Many excellent detailed books on operative surgery are available and this text is not advocated as an alternative. It is intended to facilitate revision.

Controversial issues have been avoided wherever possible. Further information should be obtained from experienced surgeons, their articles or the detailed text books.

I should like to thank Mr. A. G. Young and Mr. A. E. J. Mullins, who checked the entire book, Mr. T. G. Illtyd James of Central Middlesex Hospital, who so kindly advised on the Neurosurgical section, and the following Consultants to the Hitchin Hospitals: Mr. G. C. W. James, Mr. P. R. N. Kerr, Mr. P. Timmis, and Mr. D. W. James for their advice on various specialties.

J.J.S.

August 1962

This book has been revised; the chapter on Neurosurgery by Mr. T. G. Illtyd James, General Orthopaedics by Mr. J. M. Lancaster, and the Thorax by Mr. G. C. W. James.

My thanks are also due to Mr. J. A. Wattie who checked the entire book.

J.J.S.

January 1969

INTRODUCTION TO THE THIRD EDITION

A further revision of this book has been made. Various operations have been added including Highly Selective Vagotomy, Right Hepatic Lobectomy, Myoplastic flaps, etc.

The Vascular and Neurosurgery sections have been brought up-to-date by Mr. Roger Armour; the Orthopaedic section by Mr. John Lancaster, and the Thorax by Mr. Brian N. Pickering.

My particular thanks are due to Mr. Martin A. Clifton and Mr. Martin G. Hoffman who corrected this edition.

May I also thank the two secretaries Mrs. Vera Holloway and Miss Ann Fitch.

J.J.S.

January 1977

CONTENTS

CHAPTER I

APPENDIX, STOMACH AND DUODENUM

1. Appendicectomy
2. Perforated Peptic Ulcer
3. Posterior Gastro-enterostomy
4. Partial Gastrectomy (Polya)
5. Partial Gastrectomy (Billroth I)
6. Trans-abdominal Vagotomy
7. Highly Selective Vagotomy
8. Pyloroplasty
9. Fredet-Rammstedt's Pyloromyotomy
10. Treatment of Carcinoma of the Stomach
11. Devine's Pyloric Exclusion
12. Heller's Operation
13. Transabdominal Total Gastrectomy
14. Total Gastrectomy with Block Dissection
15. Gastrostomy
16. Re-gastrectomy for Anastomotic Ulcer

1. THE TREATMENT OF ACUTE APPENDICITIS

The treatment of acute appendicitis is appendicectomy performed after adequate resuscitation. Children in particular are carefully resuscitated; death during or immediately after operation may occur if this therapy is not carried out.

What approach is employed?
It depends on:

i. How ill the patient appears. The more the infection has affected the patient, the larger the incision.

ii. The duration. The longer the condition has been left, the larger the incision.

iii. The site. The point of maximum tenderness or the position of the caecum felt under anaesthesia affords a guide to its site. Remember two out of three are behind the caecum and the other one may be towards the midline or in the pelvis.

 The grid-iron is employed for the interval appendicectomy and should be used in the acute case only by the experienced operator, or if the inflammation does not appear to be severe.

iv. A doubtful diagnosis. In this case, a paramedian incision should be employed or the grid-iron exposure used initially as a diagnostic method.

 An abscess is drained through an incision made over its centre.

Type of incision:

i. The grid-iron approach, a transverse skin incision is used. The external oblique aponeurosis may be divided in line with a transverse skin crease incision which facilitates its extension medially into the rectus sheath. If the rectus sheath is opened and the rectus muscle is mobilised medially, the inferior epigastric vessels must be looked for and ligated. Full use is made of the muscle split from the lateral margin of rectus to the iliac spine or crest. It is made higher in children because the caecum is usually found at a higher level; if lateral extension is required the muscles are divided upwards and laterally.

 Ascending branches of the circumflex iliac artery are dealt with.

ii. The muscle cutting incision. This oblique incision is made parallel to and 2·5 cm above the inguinal ligament and sufficiently far from the iliac crest to leave a muscle fringe which will hold sutures. It is made small at the commencement and enlarged if necessary. The muscles are divided in line with the incision. This incision takes longer to sew up but affords good access.

iii. The paramedian incision is good for the pelvic appendix, but is bad for a high retrocaecal appendix. Care is taken to avoid injury to the bladder.

iv. Weir's approach. This approach is made through a transverse skin incision, through the rectus sheath and the muscles lateral to its edge. A few vessels may be found at the lateral margin of the rectus.

v. Battle's or the pararectal incision is employed by a few surgeons, but is considered unwise as nerve damage is difficult to avoid so predisposing to herniae.

Appendicectomy

i. The incision is made and the peritoneum exposed.

ii. The peritoneal cavity is opened and explored. The presence of gas and free fluid is noted. A swab for bacteriology may be taken.

iii. The appendix is found by visualisation, the exploring finger; following down the taenia coli of the caecum or by following the small bowel distally.

iv. Preferably the caecum, terminal ileum and appendix are delivered outside the wound. The first 1·5 m of the terminal ileum and its mesentery may be examined.

v. The appendix mesentery is divided to free the appendix.

vi. The appendix area is packed off.

vii. A purse-string suture is introduced around the appendix base.

viii. The appendix base is lightly crushed and ligated. An artery forceps is applied 1 cm distal to the ligation.

ix. The appendix is divided distal to the ligation and proximal to the clamp with or without cauterisation of the exposed stump mucosa.

x. The stump is inverted into the caecum and the purse-string suture is tied. Care is taken to avoid narrowing the ileum by this procedure.

xi. A check is made for haemostasis, the swabs are checked, the caecum is returned, and the wound is closed.

Helpful suggestions

i. If difficulties are encountered the incision should be enlarged immediately, erring on the side of too large an incision rather than too small. Better to repair the anterior abdominal wall than injure the bowel, or cause an ileus.

ii. Undue pulling and retracting shocks the patient more than enlarging the incision.

iii. Do not attempt to pull the appendix out of the wound – it is easier to bring out the caecum and terminal ileum. Follow the anterior taenia coli to find the appendix.

iv. The Trendelenburg or lateral tilt may help the exposure. Access may be improved by operating from the opposite side.

v. Remove in retrograde fashion.

2. THE TREATMENT OF PERFORATED PEPTIC ULCER

The perforation is closed with or without biopsy, with omental cover after adequate resuscitation. Conservative treatment is usually limited to the old and ill, particularly after 24 hours.

Partial gastrectomy is performed occasionally, if surgeon is capable, patient is fit, and with suitable indication – e.g. large perforation.

Operation

Gastric suction, drip and a suitable antibiotic are used.

i. A mid-line incision is made.

ii. Take out pyloric antrum and ask assistant to hold it.

iii. Close perforation with catgut sutures, omentum or both – take care not to narrow the lumen, introduce sutures longitudinally.

iv. Empty the peritoneal cavity of infected fluid by suction.

v. A transverse extension may be made if a high gastric ulcer is discovered, to facilitate access.

vi. Close linea alba with non-absorbable material.

3. POSTERIOR GASTRO-ENTEROSTOMY

i. A Ryle's tube is *in situ.*

ii. A left paramedian incision is made.

iii. Draw the great omentum upwards to display the transverse mesocolon to consider the practicability of establishing a retrocolic or antecolic anastomosis. Retrocolic is preferred and is described.

iv. Identify the middle colic and marginal vessels and open the mesocolon on the left of the main artery.

v. Seize the greater and lesser curvatures of the stomach with tissue forceps and draw the stomach through the opening.

vi. Rotate the forceps anti-clockwise – the greater curve then moves to the right.

vii. Approximate the edges of the hole in the mesocolon to the stomach so that the union will be clear of the anastomosis.

viii. Bring up a short loop of jejunum.

ix. Apply intestinal clamps so that the distal end of the jejunal loop lies opposite to the greater curvature.

x. Establish the anastomosis in two layers, one haemostatic, the other seromuscular.

xi. Check the afferent loop is not under tension. Make certain there are no peritoneal holes left.

4. PARTIAL GASTRECTOMY (POLYA)

i. General anaesthesia, Ryles tube and intravenous drip are required.

ii. A vertical or transverse incision is made. For gastric ulcer, incise on the left, for duodenal, on the right, or through the mid-line.

iii. Open the peritoneum and explore.

iv. There are five major parts to the operation:

(a) Mobilise the greater curvature of the stomach and preserve the middle colic vessels and mesocolon. Excise three quarters of the stomach.

(b) Mobilise all aspects of the first portion of the duodenum, ligating the right gastric artery.

(c) Divide and close the duodenum with two layers of sutures.

(d) Ligate and divide the left gastric vessels.

(e) Bring up a short loop of the first part of the jejunum and anastomose it to the divided stomach, usually afferent to the lesser curve.

v. Other points:

(a) Carefully clear the stomach at the proposed site for anastomosis.

(b) When dissecting the duodenum, keep close to it.

(c) The results with antecolic or retrocolic anastomoses are similar; antecolic are easier to dismantle and are therefore advised.

(d) The afferent loop of jejunum is kept as short as possible. The afferent loop may be fixed to the colon with a suture to prevent internal strangulations (Stammers).

(e) An adherent gastric ulcer may be pinched off the pancreas with the fingers.

(f) The upper part of the divided stomach may be closed to form a valve (Hoffmeister).

Five alternative points with a difficult duodenal dissection:

i. Attempt by careful dissection to get beyond the ulcer and sufficient duodenum to obtain a two-layered closure.

ii. Employ Bancroft-Plenk procedure of coring out the mucosa of the pyloric antrum. The problem here is that the mucosa may split into the ulcer. It is hard to be sure that all the antral mucosa has been removed. The blood supply to the remaining muscle must be preserved.

iii. Attempt closure of the duodenum by suturing the anterior duodenal wall on to the ulcer (Nissen's procedure).

iv. Suture a tube into the duodenum, bring it out through a stab wound, and aspirate continuously.

v. Divide the stomach proximal to the duodenum and close the distal portion. Dissect out the ulcer and pyloric antrum at a second stage.

5. PARTIAL GASTRECTOMY (BILLROTH I)

For Gastric Ulcer

i. Mobilise the greater curvature.

ii. Dissect out the first part of the duodenum.

iii. Divide the duodenum and keep it closed with a non-crushing clamp.

iv. Divide the left gastric vessels.

v. Divide the stomach, leaving approximately one-fifth. Close the upper part of it, leaving an aperture the size of the duodenum adjacent to the greater curvature, and approximate it to the duodenum with two layers of sutures.

vi. Close the superior duodenogastric angle with a "dangerous angle stitch". This suture takes a bite first of the anterior wall of the stomach, then the posterior layer, and finally the superior aspect of the duodenum. If possible, this suture may be repeated at a higher level as an additional safeguard.

vii. Mobilise the second part of the duodenum if any suspicion of tension is present.

6. TRANSABDOMINAL VAGOTOMY

This operation is most commonly employed in association with a gastro-enterostomy or pyloroplasty for duodenal ulcer.

i. A Ryle's tube is present in the stomach; this helps to define the oesophagus.

ii. A high left paramedian incision is made.

iii. Explore and ensure the practicability of the procedure; extensive subphrenic adhesions, if found, may make the operation difficult or unwise.

iv. Mobilise the left lobe of the liver by dividing its coronary ligament and pack it off to the right; introduce retractors on the right and left.

v. Divide the peritoneum over the oesophagus transversely.

vi. Mobilise the oesophagus and encircle it with a rubber tube. By exerting traction on the tube, dissection of the surface is facilitated. Locate the anterior nerve and strip it up and down, freeing it 5·0–7·5 cm. Resect 2·5 cm of it. Similarly deal with the posterior vagus nerve which lies away from the oesophagus and to the right. Dissect off and divide every suspicious structure on the oesophagus.

vii. Repair any hiatal defect.

7. HIGHLY SELECTIVE VAGOTOMY

i. Open the abdomen and explore.

ii. A suture is placed on the anterior surface of the lesser curvature of the stomach, 5 cm from the pylorus. This demarcates the distal level of the denervation of the stomach.

iii. The lesser omentum is examined. Identify the anterior nerve of Latarjet if possible and mark it with stay sutures to preserve the nerve during the following procedure. It is useful to identify similarly the anterior and posterior vagi at the level of the oesophagus.

iv. An opening is made in the lesser omentum on its right aspect through a bloodless area. The fingers of the left hand can then be introduced into the lesser sac to push into prominence the junction between the lesser omentum and the lesser curve of the stomach. Later a tape can be introduced around the partially mobilised lesser omentum to produce a similar effect.

v. The lesser omentum is now freed completely from the stomach between the nerve and the lesser curve. It consists of two layers and these may be divided separately. The nerves of Latarjet are carefully conserved.

vi. The dissection continues as high as the oesophagus where both vagi are preserved and the surfaces of the oesophagus are cleared of all branches as far as the hiatus.

vii. The lesser curve is inspected for ischaemic areas and re-peritonealised by seromuscular sutures.

8. PYLOROPLASTY

i. The pyloric muscle only may be divided longitudinally or the full thickness of the wall is transected longitudinally and the opening closed transversely in two layers, or in one layer and covered with omentum.

ii. Judd advocated excising any anterior ulcer present, a portion of the sphincter and pyloric antrum longitudinally, and suturing the gap transversely.

9. PYLOROMYOTOMY – FREDET RAMMSTEDT'S OPERATION

The infant is secured on a padded cross. A fine tube should be in the stomach, which has been washed out and emptied.

i. Local or general anaesthesia may be employed.

ii. A mid-line incision is relatively bloodless, or a high right rectus-splitting incision is made.

iii. The abdomen is opened and the pyloric tumour only is brought out of the wound employing two non-toothed dissecting forceps. The tumour is held firmly with the left index finger and thumb.*

iv. An incision is made longitudinally through the tumour superficially and deepened with the handle of the knife. The remaining muscle is separated widely, employing Dennis

Brown's forceps. Wide, slow and gentle opening will split the requisite amount of tissue. The mucosa is seen bulging along the length of the opening. Squeeze the stomach to ensure there is no perforation.*

v. The peritoneum is sutured and the rectus sheath approximated with interrupted sutures.

vi. The child is taken off the cross and placed on its side to avoid accidental inhalation.*

vii. Feeding is commenced immediately.

10. TREATMENT OF CARCINOMA OF STOMACH

There are "five" surgical treatments of this condition:

i. Radical or palliative partial gastrectomy. Proximal or distal gastrectomy.

ii. Total gastrectomy with or without block dissection.

iii. Palliative gastrojejunostomy.

iv. Devine's pyloric exclusion operation.

v. Gastrostomy or jejunostomy.

11. DEVINE'S PYLORIC EXCLUSION (PALLIATIVE PROCEDURE)

The purpose of the operation is to exclude an obstructing and necrotic tumour of distal part of stomach.

i. An intravenous drip and Ryle's tube are required.

ii. Mobilise the uninvolved area of the stomach by dividing structures along both curves.

iii. Divide the stomach.

* Points requiring particular notice are marked with an asterisk throughout.

iv. Close the distal end carefully in two layers.

v. Anastomose first loop of jejunum to proximal cut end of stomach.

vi. Close abdomen carefully to avoid wound dehiscence.

12. OESOPHAGO-CARDIOMYOTOMY

Heller's Operation

i. A Ryle's tube is present in stomach.

ii. A high left paramedian incision is made (or a thoracotomy may be used).

iii. The abdomen is opened and explored.

iv. The left hepatic lobe is drawn down and its coronary ligament divided.

v. The peritoneum is divided over the oesophagus.

vi. The oesophagus is mobilised and a rubber tube introduced around it to act as a retractor.

vii. A longitudinal incision about 10 cm long is now made through the anterior wall of the oesophagus, cardia and body of stomach to expose the mucosa. All fibres are carefully divided. The vagi are preserved.

viii. Haemostasis is secured. The stomach is compressed to reveal any leaks. Any defect at the hiatus is repaired.

ix. The rubber sling is removed.

x. The abdomen is closed.

13. TRANSABDOMINAL TOTAL GASTRECTOMY

i. A drip and Ryle's tube are *in situ*.

ii. A long left paramedian incision is made.

iii. Open the peritoneum and explore.

iv. Mobilise the greater curvature up to the oesophagus.

v. Mobilise all aspects of the first part of the duodenum, divide and close it.

vi. Divide the left gastric and extend the division of the lesser omentum as far as the oesophagus. This manoeuvre is aided by mobilising the left lobe of the liver by dividing the coronary ligament.

vii. A loop of jejunum is brought up either in front of, or behind, the colon, and anastomosed to the oesophagus in two layers behind the stomach, which is amputated only when the anastomosis is nearly completed. The mucosa is the strong layer in the oesophagus.* To avoid "drag" suture the anastomosis to its surroundings.

viii. The anastomosis easily leaks and great care should be employed in forming this anastomosis. It is performed in two layers with non-absorbable material. Alternatively a Roux en Y procedure may be used.

ix. A side-to-side anastomosis is made in the jejunal loop (Braun).

x. The Ryle's tube may be left in, either with its tip just above the anastomosis, or through it.

14. TOTAL GASTRECTOMY WITH BLOCK DISSECTION

i. In addition to the above procedure, the greater omentum is stripped off the transverse colon and removed with the stomach.

ii. The lesser omentum is removed as completely as possible.

iii. The spleen and the tail and part of the body of the pancreas is mobilised by drawing the spleen to the right and dividing the peritoneum behind it with a long scissors. The spleen and that portion of the pancreas can thus be mobilised by digital dissection and removed with the stomach.

iv. The splenic vessels are ligated, the pancreas cut across and its raw end closed with interrupted linen or silk sutures.

15. GASTROSTOMY

i. Local or general anaesthesia is employed.

ii. A high left vertical muscle-splitting incision is made. Note that the stomach rises high when it is empty.

iii. Bring the stomach out of the wound and hold its anterior surface with tissue forceps. Pack off the area.

iv. Insert a purse-string suture and make an aperture through its centre to open the stomach.

v. Insert a 12 or 14 Jacques catheter, then anchor it to the stomach with a linen suture.

vi. Close with two purse-string sutures around the catheter.

vii. Test the tube and the closure of the stomach about it, with sterile water and a funnel.

viii. Close the wound and fix the tube to the skin.

ix. If the tube accidentally comes out, it must be replaced immediately.

16. RE-GASTRECTOMY FOR ANASTOMOTIC ULCER

i. Ryle's tube and intravenous drip are in position.

ii. The abdomen is opened through one of the original incisions and the anterior abdominal wall is cleared of adhesions by sharp dissection.

iii. The wound may be extended to the left by a horizontal cut made below the costal margin.

iv. The stomach is mobilised along the greater curvature to the oesophagus.

v. The efferent and afferent loops of jejunum should be exposed and the mesocolon with its middle colic vessels is identified.

vi. A search is made for the ulcer, and the stomach may be opened if it is not identified externally.

vii. A cause is sought, such as a pancreatic adenoma,* or a pyloric antrum not previously excised. Either is removed if found. A vagotomy is performed if intact fibres are found.*

viii. The stomach and jejunal loop are now fully mobilised and detached from the mesocolon.

ix. A further portion of stomach, anastomosis and half-inch of jejunum on either side are now removed.

x. The jejunum is now reunited.

xi. A new anastomosis is made between the jejunum and remaining portion of stomach, distal to the anastomosis just performed.

xii. The hole is repaired in the mesocolon or is re-affixed to the stomach for retrocolic anastomosis.

CHAPTER II

SMALL AND LARGE BOWEL

17. Principles in Management of Intestinal Obstruction
18. Small Intestine Anastomosis
19. Intussusception
20. Jejunostomy
21. Surgery of the Colon
22. Caecostomies
23. Ileostomy
24. Transverse Colostomy
25. Right Hemicolectomy
26. Left Hemicolectomy
27. Total Colectomy
28. Excision Pelvic Colon
29. Restorative Resection of Rectum
30. Abdominal Dissection of Abdominoperineal Excision of Rectum
31. Perineal Dissection of Abdominoperineal Excision of Rectum
32. Rectosigmoidectomy for Hirschsprung's Disease
33. Treatment of Rectal Prolapse

17. MANAGEMENT OF ACUTE INTESTINAL OBSTRUCTION

General principles

i. Perform a laparotomy as soon as resuscitation permits. It is impossible to exclude strangulation.*

ii. A Ryle's tube and an intravenous drip are required. A straight X-ray of the abdomen is in Theatre.

iii. A further rectal examination, sigmoidoscopy,* and examination of the abdomen under anaesthesia may be helpful.

iv. Open the abdomen, observe the presence of free fluid, or gas.

v. The caecum is examined for distension.

vi. Collapsed and distended loops are traced to the obstruction site.

vii. If possible exteriorisation of a complicated obstruction should be carried out. The cause may then be seen and the appropriate method of relief decided upon.

viii. Suction of the foul fluid above an obstruction with a modified sucker (Savage), prevents its sudden absorption and consequent circulatory collapse that may follow the release of the strangulation. Furthermore the closure of the abdomen is facilitated and ileus may be avoided.

ix. Great gentleness is used in handling the bowel particularly if peritonitis is present. The surgical procedures are reduced to the minimum necessary to restore function.

18. SMALL INTESTINE ANASTOMOSIS

i. The mesentery is always divided first – in malignant cases a large V-section has to be taken in order to incorporate any glandular spread. In other cases less mesentery is excised.

ii. Place the line of transection in healthy bowel well proximal to the diseased or distended bowel or leakage may occur.*

iii. Clear the entire bowel circumference from the mesentery at the site of anastomosis for just less than 5 mm – no more – so that fat does not obscure the edges and make anastomosis difficult.

iv. Soft intestinal clamps are applied 4 cm from the ends, they occlude the lumen, but must not compress the mesentery.

v. Check the position of the mesenteries.

vi. There must be no tension on the suture line attachment.*

vii. Stay sutures facilitate suturing.

viii. The "through and through" continuous haemostatic catgut suture is introduced first and then the continuous seromuscular suture. Lock the posterior layer of the "through and through" suture to avoid narrowing.

ix. Repair the hole in mesentery.

19. INTUSSUSCEPTION

i. An intravenous drip, Ryle's tube and an empty bladder are necessary.

ii. A lower right (rectus-splitting) paramedian incision is made.

iii. The abdomen is opened and by employing two fingers inside* the peritoneal cavity, the intussusception is reduced as far as the caecum.

iv. The caecum is now brought out of the wound and the last part of the reduction performed under vision.

v. The bowel is examined following the reduction for perforation or gangrenous areas.

vi. If reduction is difficult, gentle pressure is exerted on the apex of the intussusception over a moist pack.

vii. If the reduction is very difficult, avoid waiting too long, which shocks the child (and may tear the bowel) and proceed directly with resection and anastomosis.

viii. An alternative procedure is described by Woodhall: The intussusception is resected and a side-to-side ileo-transverse anastomosis is made 5 cm from the clamped ends. The clamped ends are brought out through the wound and a week later when the bowel is functioning, an extraperitoneal closure of the ends is performed. Ileal distension can be relieved by temporary removal of the clamp.

20. JEJUNOSTOMY

i. An upper vertical left rectus-splitting incision is made.

ii. The duodenal-jejunal junction is identified and a loop of bowel approximately 45 cm distal to it is brought out through the wound. The area is packed off. Intestinal clamps are applied at each end.

iii. Two stay-sutures are inserted at either end of the loop on the antimesenteric border.

iv. A longitudinal cut 5 cm long is made down to the mucosa, and a small opening made at its distal end into which is inserted a No. 9 Jacques catheter. It is fixed at this opening with a suture which runs through the wall of the tube.

v. The catheter is then allowed to lie in the trough thus made, and is covered by interrupted sutures of catgut.

vi. The clamps are removed and the tube is then tested by running in sterile water.

vii. The tube is then threaded through the greater omentum and brought out through the main or separate stab wound.

viii. The bowel is dropped back after which the tube is carefully anchored to the skin*, and the wound is closed.

Five dangers

i. If the tube is pushed too far in, the bowel may be perforated by pressure from its tip.

ii. The lumen may be narrowed by excessive suturing and intestinal obstruction may result.

iii. The tube may come out causing peritonitis (it is equivalent to a high intestinal perforation and must be replaced immediately).

iv. If the tube is too large, it may obstruct the lumen, and an intestinal fistula may result.

v. As it is handled four-hourly, it may easily be pulled out. It must be fixed securely to the skin.

21. SURGERY OF THE COLON

Five general principles

i. Prepare bowel by using low-residue or elemental diets, clearing the bowel content by using enemas, wash-outs and purgation, and using intestinal antibiotics.

ii. In the presence of acute intestinal obstruction and an ill patient, minimal surgery is undertaken.

iii. Operations for cancer must have adequate resections.

iv. Confirm that the edges of the bowel are adequately vascularised by the appearance, and bleeding from the edges.

v. Prevent tension on the suture line by adequate mobilisation: the structures are brought into apposition and are not sutured tightly to one another.

Elective Surgery for the Various Carcinoma Sites

i. For carcinoma of the right colon, perform a right hemicolectomy; take more of the transverse colon and its mesentery if the growth is situated at the hepatic flexure site.

ii. Carcinoma of the transverse colon is treated by excision of the transverse colon and the appropriate mesentery.

iii. Carcinoma of the left colon is treated by left hemicolectomy.

The Treatment of Acute Obstruction Arising from these Various Sites

i. Obstructing carcinoma of the right colon is treated by an ileo-transverse colostomy. If the colon is distended due to a competent ileocaecal valve, a caecostomy must be established as well, to avoid perforation, or a right hemicolectomy is performed.

ii. Obstruction of the hepatic flexure is relieved similarly, but place the entero-anastomosis well over to the left of the transverse colon.

iii. Obstruction of the transverse colon may be treated by a caecostomy or by excising the growth with its mesentery and bringing out the remaining bowel loops as a spur colostomy, or immediate resection and anastomosis is undertaken. This latter operation is only performed if the patient is fit, the operation is easy, and the surgeon competent.

iv. Obstruction of the splenic flexure is treated by a caecostomy or by a colostomy well proximal to the growth. This may necessitate mobilisation of the hepatic flexure, but will facilitate the ultimate anastomosis.

v. Obstruction of the descending colon is treated similarly by hepatic-flexure colostomy.

vi. Obstruction of the pelvic colon is also treated by hepatic flexure colostomy.

Alternatively with malignant obstructions of the left colon, resect the growth and its mesentery, establish the proximal cut end of the bowel as a colostomy, close the distal end and return it to the abdomen.

Restoration of the continuity of the bowel is undertaken as a second stage (Sames) or, if patient's condition is satisfactory, perform definitive operation of radical excision and anastomosis.

22. CAECOSTOMY

Exteriorising Part of Caecum

This method tends to be safer; however, it is not popular and requires formal closure.

i. A muscle-cutting incision is made over the caecum.

ii. The caecum is brought out of the wound and a Paul's tube inserted into it and held in place by an encircling ligature.

iii. The wound is closed with interrupted sutures. The caecal wall is sutured only to the skin. If fixed more deeply, a faecal fistula may result.

Blind Caecostomy

i. Muscle-cutting or grid-iron incision is made over the caecum.

ii. Part of the caecum is brought out of the wound. Great care is required as it may split.

iii. Stay sutures are introduced. Two concentric purse-string sutures are inserted and the bowel opened – it may be emptied by employing Savage's intestinal sucker. A large De Pezzer catheter with its cone-end partially removed is inserted and the purse-strings drawn together.

iv. The caecum and tube are then returned to the abdomen and the wound closed.

v. Wash through tube daily to avoid blockage.

23. ILEOSTOMY

i. Five points regarding its site:

(a) Not too near the umbilicus.

(b) Not too near the groin; too much movement may displace the bag.

(c) Not too near a wound. Subsequent scarring of the wound may draw in the ileostomy and distort it.

(d) Not too near a bony point; the problem of fixing apparatus arises.

(e) Not too low or too near the waistline, the more conspicuous the apparatus becomes.

ii. Make a right lower vertical trans-rectus incision.

iii. Identify the ileum entering the caecum.

iv. The ileal mesentery is examined and divided approximately 5 cm from the bowel, preserving the leash of vessels which supplies the ileostomy.

v. "Trephine" a hole say 5 cm to the right and just below the level of the umbilicus. Insert a Parker-Kerr forcep through the opening and clamp it on the ileum. Clamp the ileum again distally, pack off the area, then divide the bowel. Bring the clamped ileum out through the trephined opening. The lateral space may be closed or the ileal mesentery edge sutured to the parietal peritoneum.

vi. Close the distal end of the ileum with two layers of sutures.

vii. Remove the pack; close and seal off the main wound.

viii. Remove the clamp from the bowel and suture the open end of the ileostomy to the skin with interrupted sutures to form a spout 2·5 to 3·8 cm long. Haemostasis is obtained.

ix. Apply ileostomy apparatus.

24. TRANSVERSE COLOSTOMY WITH SPUR

i. Incision – a vertical trans-rectus 8 cm long with two-thirds of the incision above the umbilicus.

ii. Exploration – find the transverse colon by following up the great omentum.

iii. Withdraw the transverse colon. During this procedure prevent other parts of the bowel emerging.

iv. Draw the great omentum upwards and dissect it off* the colon by small cuts with knife and scissors. Tie any bleeding vessels.

v. Make a hole in the mesentery close to the bowel.

vi. Push through a glass rod held at one end by a piece of rubber tubing.

vii. Approximate the nearest taeniae of the afferent and efferent loops over 10 cm or more with interrupted sutures to form an adequate spur.

viii. Close the peritoneum and rectus sheath and skin with interrupted sutures, leaving room for one finger only beside the bowel.

ix. Do not fix the wall of the bowel to the peritoneum owing to the danger of causing a faecal fistula. It may permissible to attach the peritoneum to the appendices epiploicae.

x. Pack off the area.

xi. Open the colostomy by making an incision 5 cm long; tie off any bleeding vessels.

25. RIGHT HEMICOLECTOMY

i. An intravenous drip and Ryle's tube are in position, and an indwelling catheter is employed.

ii. A long right paramedian incision is made.

iii. Open the peritoneum and explore.

iv. Pack off the intestine to the left.

v. Dissect the great omentum off the right side of the transverse colon to expose the hepatic flexure, or divide a portion of it and remove it with the right colon.

vi. Mobilise the ascending colon by dividing the peritoneum along its right margin. Mobilise the hepatic flexure and terminal ileum.

vii. Bring the colon, its mesentery and terminal ileum out of the abdomen by blunt dissection behind these structures; avoid damaging the duodenum, ureter, ovarian or spermatic vessels.

viii. Decide on the site of division of the terminal ileum and the transverse colon. At least 15 cm of the ileum are removed as the blood supply of this segment may be reduced by the division of the ileocolic vessels. The right colic, ileocolic and the marginal branch of the transverse colon are divided with the mesentery. The origin of the main vessels are seen arising from the superior mesenteric artery.

ix. The area is packed off and the right colon and ileum clamped and divided at each end and the intervening bowel removed.

x. The ileum is then anastomosed to the transverse colon (end-to-end, end-to-side, side-to-end or side-to-side).

xi. The lumen of the ileum may be increased in size by dividing the bowel obliquely.

xii. A two-layered anastomosis is performed. In view of the slow healing of the colon, due to its poor blood supply, one layer of sutures of non-absorbable material is used.

xiii. The gap in the mesentery is closed.

xiv. The packs are removed.

xv. No attempt is made to cover the raw area.

26. LEFT HEMICOLECTOMY

i. A drip, Ryle's tube and catheter are in position.

ii. A long left paramedian incision is made.

iii. The peritoneum is opened and explored.

iv. The bowel is packed to the right to expose the left colon.

v. The left colon is mobilised by dividing the peritoneal attachments on the left as far as the splenic flexure.

vi. A variable part of the great omentum may be excised with the transverse colon depending on the site of the growth.

vii. The transverse colon is mobilised as far as the splenic flexure.

viii. The splenic flexure is then mobilised. (The paramedian incision is extended transversely or obliquely to the left if difficulty with this last procedure is encountered.)

ix. A V-shaped area of mesentery is now divided including the left colic and if necessary the middle colic vessels.

x. The area is packed off and the left colon removed.

xi. An end-to-end two-layered anastomosis is made between the transverse and pelvic colons.

xii. The opening in the mesentery is then repaired.

xiii. The pack is removed.

27. TOTAL COLECTOMY

i. A drip, Ryle's tube and catheter are in position.

ii. A long left paramedian incision is employed.

iii. The bowel is mobilised as in a right and left hemicolectomy. The mesentery is divided.

iv. The area is packed off, the ileum is divided obliquely and is anastomosed to the rectum as an end-to-end or side-to-side anastomosis, or end-to-side, or brought out as an ileostomy.

v. The gap in the mesentery is closed.

vi. The abdomen is closed.

28. EXCISION OF PELVIC COLON

i. A Ryle's tube is in the stomach; a catheter lies in the bladder, which is emptied.

ii. A lower left paramedian incision is employed.

iii. The peritoneum is opened and explored.

iv. The pelvic colon is held and the rest of the bowel packed away.

v. A self-retaining retractor is inserted.

vi. The pelvic colon is mobilised by dividing the congenital adhesions on its lateral aspect.

vii. The left ureter,* and ovarian or testicular vessels, are clearly seen or found by division of the peritoneum and dissection.

viii. The mesentery is examined and the sites for division of the bowel decided, so that the ends may be brought together subsequently without tension.

ix. The mesentery is now divided.

x. Clamps are applied and the segment of bowel is removed.

xi. The bowel ends are anastomosed with two layers of sutures.

xii. Any peritoneal holes are obliterated.

xiii. The wound is closed.

29. RESTORATIVE RESECTION OF RECTUM

Five points to be considered

i. The growth should be beyond reach of a rectal examination with a finger, that is, above 10 cm.

ii. On biopsy examination, the growth should not be highly anaplastic.

iii. The patient should not be too fat.

iv. The patient's pelvis should be normal or wide.

v. If secondaries are found in the liver, this type of operation is preferable, if the other conditions are fulfilled.

i. A Ryle's tube, an intravenous drip and catheter are placed in position.

ii. A long left paramedian incision is made.

iii. The abdomen is opened and explored. After examining the blood supply of the mesocolon and the growth, the sites for the division of the colon and rectum are decided.

iv. The pelvic colon is held and the rest of the bowel packed away.

v. The table is tilted into the Trendelenburg position if it aids exposure, and a self-retaining retractor placed in the wound.

vi. The pelvic colon is partly freed by dividing the congenital adhesions on its lateral aspect.

vii. The amount of peritoneum of pelvic floor to be removed with the growth is now demarcated by dividing it with a knife or scissors; the incision runs from the colon at the proposed site of division laterally over the mesocolon, anteriorly across the base of the bladder or region of cervix 12 mm in front of the lowest point of the peritoneal floor,* then upwards on the medial side of the mesocolon, returning to the original level.

viii. The peritoneum of the pelvis is now raised by sharp and blunt dissection to expose the ureters* and ovarian or testicular vessels.

ix. Commencing at the proposed site for division of the colon, the mesocolon is divided down to its root.

x. The main pedicle containing the superior haemorrhoidal vessels is dissected free and after ensuring that both ureters are safe, ligated and divided.

xi. The rectosigmoid mesentery is now freed from the sacrum by a few cuts with the scissors, and by digital dissection posterior to it the fascia of Waldeyer may be reached posterior to the rectum. The dissection anterior to the rectum is now commenced; the seminal vesicles or vaginal wall are identified.

xii. By division of bands behind the seminal vesicles or vaginal wall, the fascia of Denonvilliers is opened and a plane of dissection found leading down to the apex of the prostate or the perineal body.

xiii. The lateral ligaments containing the middle haemorrhoidal vessels are now ligated and divided.

xiv. The site for the proposed division of the rectum is now fixed by dividing the mesorectum. The bowel wall is cleared of fat.

xv. A right-angled clamp is now placed over the rectum, and the rectum may be washed out.

xvi. Crushing clamps are now placed above and below, and the diseased bowel and its mesentery removed.

xvii. The end of the colon is now anastomosed to the upper end of the rectum using one or two layers of sutures.

xviii. The horizontal mattress sutures of non-absorbable material attain their greatest value in this difficult anastomosis (Grey Turner).

xix. The floor of the peritoneum is closed.

xx. The wound is closed. An intra- or extra-peritoneal drain may be left in.

30. ABDOMINAL DISSECTION OF ABDOMINO-PERINEAL EXCISION OF RECTUM

The dissection proceeds as described in i-xiii of Restorative Resection of Rectum.

31. PERINEAL DISSECTION OF ABDOMINO-PERINEAL EXCISION OF RECTUM

i. The patient is in the lithotomy-Trendelenburg position, employing the Lloyd-Davies' apparatus.

ii. The bladder is emptied and a catheter left in.

iii. A sandbag or "rest" under the sacrum facilitates the approach to the coccyx.

iv. The anus is closed with two purse-string sutures.

v. An encircling incision is made around the anus, extending over the coccyx.

vi. The incision is deepened through the perianal space and fascia into the ischiorectal fossa.

vii. The coccyx is identified and a portion of it freed by inserting a knife through one of its articulations.

viii. This division is extended on both sides so that a finger may be introduced around the ileococcygeus to facilitate its division.

ix. The inferior haemorrhoidal vessels are ligated.

x. A self-retaining retractor is inserted.

xi. The fascia of Waldeyer posterior to the rectum is now divided.

xii. The tissues are divided anterior to the rectum, keeping behind the transverse perineal muscles.

xiii. Avoiding the mid-line, the pubococcygeus muscle is divided.

xiv. The prostate and urethra with its catheter are now identified and by further careful division, the plane of Denonvilliers is entered, lying behind the prostate. The bowel turns sharply backwards at the anorectal junction and the dissection must follow this line to avoid urethral damage. The abdominal surgeon assists in defining the tissue planes.

xv. The lateral ligaments are ligated and divided.

xvi. With anterior growths, the whole posterior portion of the vagina is excised.

xvii. The perineal wound is closed with drainage, and if necessary packed with gauze.

xviii. The vaginal orifice is re-formed.

32. RECTO-SIGMOIDECTOMY FOR HIRSCHSPRUNG'S DISEASE

If a previous colostomy has been required to relieve obstruction, the proposed site for subsequent division of the bowel is marked with black sutures 12 cm proximal to the "cone".* Following the colostomy the bowel distal to it collapses, and the affected segment is no longer identifiable.

Operation

i. General anaesthesia, modified lithotomy-Trendelenburg position, catheter and Ryle's tube are required.

ii. Anterior resection and anastomosis is performed through a lower left paramedian incision, but the rectum is "cored out" by keeping close to it, thereby avoiding damage to the pelvic nerves.

iii. If the anastomosis is too deep, a pull-through abdomino-anal technique (Swenson) may be employed.

iv. The resection and anastomosis of the bowel may be performed outside the anus. A sigmoidoscope is passed, two 35 cm long needles carrying the ends of thread looped on the bowel are then inserted through the instrument from above. The sigmoidoscope is removed and by traction on the threads, the bowel is prolapsed (Dennis Browne).

v. The pelvic peritoneum and anterior abdominal wall are then repaired with or without an extraperitoneal drain.

vi. The peritoneal cavity extension around the inner loop of bowel is opened by dividing the outer layer of the prolapse.

vii. The inner tube of bowel is pulled down until the marker sutures appear.

viii. The two layers are then divided transversely and sutured together with interrupted sutures.

ix. To avoid incontinence, 19 mm of the anal canal should be left beyond the mucocutaneous junction.

33. RECTAL PROLAPSE

Thiersch Operation

Silver wire may be inserted round the anus subcutaneously to control the prolapse.

Partial Rectal Prolapse

A modified haemorrhoidectomy, i.e. excision of wedge of mucous membrane may be performed. The size of the mucosal pedicle transfixed is greater and its ligation therefore requires more care.

Roscoe Graham's Operation

General principles

It is essential to mobilise the rectum down to the anorectal ring to obtain a clear view of the puborectalis muscles so that their repair may be performed. The abnormal pouch of Douglas is excised and the pelvic floor reconstituted (Goligher).

i. The bowel has been prepared, the bladder is empty, a Ryle's tube is in the stomach and an intravenous transfusion is functioning.

ii. The patient is placed in the Trendelenburg or the lithotomy-Trendelenburg position.

iii. The abdomen is opened and explored through a long left paramedian incision.

iv. Care must be exercised throughout the procedure to preserve the ureters.

v. The pelvic colon and rectum are mobilised down to the anorectal ring. The dissection is similar to the details described for the anterior resection of the rectum except that the dissection keeps close to the rectum to avoid damaging the autonomic nerves and the superior rectal vessels are preserved.

vi. The puborectalis muscles are sutured together in front of the rectum.

vii. The redundant pouch of Douglas is excised and the pelvic peritoneal floor reconstituted.

viii. Alternatively a piece of polyvinyl sponge 7·5 cm wide ×12·5 cm long is anchored to the sacrum, wrapped around the rectum and fixed with sutures (Wells).

CHAPTER III

ANAL CANAL

34. Treatment of Perianal and Ischiorectal Abscesses
35. Excision of Fistula-in-ano
36. Sigmoidoscopy and Haemorrhoidectomy
37. Pilonidal Sinus
38. Internal Sphincterotomy for Chronic Fissure-in-ano

34. PERIANAL AND ISCHIORECTAL ABSCESS

i. General anaesthesia and the lithotomy position are employed.

ii. Digital and proctoscopic examination may then be carried out.

iii. The abscess is opened and sufficient skin removed to allow free drainage.

iv. A fistula may be found and its site marked by a ligature (seton) for attention later.

35. FISTULA-IN-ANO

i. Excise or lay open the tract and send the tissue for biopsy.

ii. The pubo-rectalis muscle at the anorectal ring must be preserved, or incontinence results.*

iii. Adequate external drainage must be established.

iv. Shallow wounds without overhanging edges should be made.

v. Lay open all other ramifications.

To Identify Continence Muscle (Pubo-rectalis)

i. It may be felt with the examining finger, but is deficient anteriorly.

ii. The patient is asked to "draw up the back passage". The muscle is felt to contract.

iii. Pass a proctoscope into the ampulla of rectum, then slowly withdraw it. The lumen closes and as it does so the site of the muscle is revealed.

iv. Pass a silver probe through the fistula; if the anal canal closes behind it, the site of the internal opening is below the muscle. If the anal canal remains open the internal opening is above the muscle.

v. If doubt exists, a thread of seton is passed through the fistula at operation. When the patient is conscious, the site of the internal opening can be felt and its relationship with the anorectal ring established.

36. SIGMOIDOSCOPY AND HAEMORRHOIDECTOMY

i. The patient is first placed on his left side, and a sigmoidoscopy is performed. The instrument is inserted and its obturator withdrawn. The rectal lumen or its edge is seen as the instrument ascends. Inflation of the rectum with air aids the view. The instrument having reached above 22 or so centimetres if possible is withdrawn and the bowel wall re-examined as the instrument is taken out.

ii. The position of the patient is changed to the lithotomy position.

iii. The perianal skin is prepared.

iv. The skin overlying the three primary haemorrhoids, that is, 4 o'clock, 7 o'clock and 11 o'clock, is grasped by artery forceps.

v. Traction is exerted on the forceps and this reveals the piles. Further forceps are applied until the pedicles are reached.

vi. An index finger is inserted into the rectum and the same hand holds the two forceps, i.e. one on the pile and one on the skin margin, and exerts traction on the pedicle and on the corresponding portion of external skin.

vii. A V-shaped portion of skin is excised and dissected up to expose the lower end of the internal sphincter.

viii. The pedicle is transfixed with catgut or silk, and the pile excised.

ix. The other two piles are dealt with in a similar fashion.

x. Other haemorrhoids are dealt with similarly, but with conservation of the skin. Adequate skin bridges are preserved.

xi. Petroleum jelly is introduced into the anal canal.

xii. A rectal tube is inserted.

xiii. Three gauzes soaked in Eusol and whose corners are lubricated with petroleum jelly are introduced around the tube so as to exert pressure on the remaining perianal skin.

xiv. Further gauzes are applied so as to build up the area around the tube.

xv. A T-bandage is applied.

Other points

i. One per cent of haemorrhoidectomies bleed postoperatively.

ii. The bowels are opened by using Milpar and a purgative given on the second night.

iii. Dilatation is carried out from the fourth day.

iv. The wounds are dressed twice a day by tucking in a moistened corner of gauze.

v. The wounds occasionally need to be touched with silver nitrate to keep down excessive granulation tissue.

37. PILONIDAL SINUS

i. General anaesthesia; a swab of any pus present is sent for culture; the bowel is prepared, the area is shaved. Injection of a dye may be helpful.

ii. The affected area is widely excised down to the sacrum.

iii. If the edges come together without tension, the defect is obliterated with sutures (Oldham). If not, the wound is packed.

iv. Buried sutures are avoided to prevent recurrence.

v. The inner layer of sutures are vertical mattress sutures and include the sacral periosteum. The outer layer are through and through, and again include the periosteum.

vi. By this procedure, the space deep to the skin may be obliterated.

vii. The bowels are confined for seven days – if possible – after the operation.

38. INTERNAL SPHINCTEROTOMY FOR CHRONIC FISSURE-IN-ANO

i. General anaesthesia is employed. Local, however, may be used.

ii. The patient is placed in the left lateral or lithotomy position, and a sigmoidoscopy is carried out.

iii. The patient is then put into the lithotomy position and the perianal skin swabbed with 1 per cent Cetrimide.

iv. A proctoscope is passed. Polyps found are excised, as are associated haemorrhoids.

v. Local anaesthetic with 1/100,000 Adrenalin is introduced under the mucosa of the anal canal in the midline posteriorly, to reduce bleeding.

vi. A few minutes are allowed to elapse, following which a rectal speculum is introduced into the anal canal and opened.

vii. A linear incision is made, starting 5 mm above the dentate line between two rectal columns, extending to just below the anus.

viii. The incision is deepened to expose the white transverse fibres of the internal sphincter, and these are divided with the scalpel until the longitudinal muscle is reached. This appears as a sheet of whitish tissue.

ix. Following this the speculum is removed and the external wound is examined. Further excision of skin is made to include the tag and in order to produce a flat, pear-shaped wound, in which no transverse bars of tissue remain.

x. Petroleum jelly is introduced into the rectum, a rectal tube is inserted followed by a flat gauze dressing soaked in Eusol.

CHAPTER IV

EXTERNAL ABDOMINAL HERNIAE

39. INGUINAL HERNIA REPAIR IN THE INFANT

i. A transverse incision is made a finger's breadth above the pubic spine.

ii. The incision is deepened through the fatty layer of Camper and the more definite layer of Scarpa down to the external oblique and the emerging cord.

iii. The routine procedure subsequently described for adults is then followed.

iv. Alternatively, the testis and hernia is gently brought out of the scrotum and the gubernaculum divided.

v. Approaching laterally the cremasteric layer and the internal spermatic fascia are divided to expose the vas deferens and spermatic veins which lie separately.

vi. The diaphanous fascia overlying the vas and veins is divided to allow complete mobilisation of these structures.

vii. With these two vital structures away, the routine mobilisation opening and excision of the sac (or its proximal part only) follows.

viii. The hole in the fascia transversalis through which the sac emerged is usually not repaired.

ix. The testis is replaced.

x. The external oblique is repaired.

xi. The skin is closed with a subcuticular catgut suture and covered with plastic dressing.

40. INGUINAL HERNIA REPAIR IN THE ADULT

Elective Case

i. General or local anaesthesia is employed. The bladder should be empty.*

ii. A transverse incision is made terminating a finger-breadth above the pubic spine or an oblique incision is drawn a finger-breadth above and parallel to the medial half of the inguinal ligament.

iii. The incision is deepened to expose the external oblique and the external ring.

iv. The external oblique is divided to expose the cord, taking care to avoid damaging the cutaneous nerves subjacent to the aponeurosis.

v. The cremaster is picked up between two artery forceps and divided and dissected back to expose the contents.

vi. An indirect sac may be found within the cord and dissected upwards to a level beyond its neck.
A direct sac may be discovered lying behind the cord. Part of the direct sac may be excised if it is large, or it may simply be pushed back and covered by the repair or invaginated employing the "Keel" repair technique. If the sac is excised care must be taken to ensure that the bladder is not opened on its medial aspect.

vii. The neck of the sac recognised by the extraperitoneal fat is now transfixed and ligated and the sac excised.

viii. The pubic spine is exposed so that repair of this area may be clearly visualised.

ix. The conjoint tendon is approximated to the inguinal ligament with interrupted or continuous sutures of non-absorbable material, being careful to close the internal ring snugly about the cord. The periosteum over the pubis is used to hold the medial suture.

x. If tension is present, Tanner's slide is performed as follows:

> The external oblique is raised over the rectus sheath, exposing the conjoint tendon.
> The conjoint tendon is incised 12 mm from the mid-line, and extended down to the pubis.
> The conjoint tendon now slides down and may be anchored with two sutures to the rectus muscle so as to prevent it descending more than the required amount.

xi. The external oblique is repaired, and the wound is closed.

41. STRANGULATED INGUINAL HERNIA

i. The same technique is followed as before, except that when the sac is reached the area is packed off to catch any infected fluid that may pour out.*

ii. The constricting agent is the peritoneal neck,* which is carefully divided under vision, a procedure that may be helped if a hernia director is employed.

iii. The bowel is examined following its release and if the colour improves, or it bleeds, or the vessels pulsate, it is returned to the abdomen. Take care that gangrenous bowel does not slip back into the main peritoneal cavity.

iv. If the bowel is gangrenous, and the access inadequate, the wound may be enlarged upwards and laterally like a Rutherford-Morison incision, and an appropriate amount of bowel for the anastomosis delivered. The mesentery of the bowel is divided and an end-to-end or side-to-side anastomosis is performed. The hole in the mesentery is repaired.

v. The removal of gangrenous bowel should not be conservative, because the area above the gangrenous portion is usually distended and its blood supply may have been affected, resulting in the subsequent breakdown of the anastomosis.

vi. The hernial defect is now repaired.

42. FEMORAL HERNIA REPAIR

(Annandale and Lotheisson) including Strangulation

i. The usual inguinal hernia incision is made, after ensuring that the bladder is empty.*

ii. The incision is then deepened and the lower skin flap mobilised and retracted to expose the femoral hernia.

iii. The sac coverings are divided and if strangulated, the area is packed off.* The peritoneal sac is then opened below and laterally, and the infected fluid removed. The bowel is held if suspect, as it tends to disappear into the abdomen during the subsequent procedure.

iv. The external oblique is divided.

v. The cord is mobilised to expose the fascia transversalis, the inferior epigastric vessels and branches, and a possible abnormal obturator artery. If necessary, the abnormal vessel is ligated.

vi. To make an opening through the fascia transversalis, a closed artery forceps is applied to the fascia and opened, the neck of the sac is then revealed.

vii. The conjoint tendon is retracted upwards to improve the exposure.

viii. The peritoneum above the neck of the sac is opened and extended down to include the neck. A hernia director is used if necessary to protect the bowel.

ix. If helpful, Lacunar Ligament is divided and rarely the inguinal ligament is divided close to the pubic spine and turned back (Hey Groves).

x. The bowel is returned or resected.

xi. The sac is brought up from below and excised. The opening in the peritoneum is closed.

xii. Taking care of the external iliac vein, the conjoint tendon is sutured to Pectineal Ligament.

xiii. The external oblique is repaired.

xiv. The wound is closed.

Femoral Hernia Repair – Low Approach (Lockwood)

i. An incision is made over the hernia, a finger-breadth below the medial half of the inguinal ligament.

ii. The incision is deepened to expose the sac and its coverings.

iii. The hernia with coverings is held and the structures surrounding it are dissected off by sharp and blunt dissection until the neck is reached.

iv. The sac is opened on its lower lateral aspect to avoid opening the bladder.

v. The sac neck is transfixed and the redundant sac excised. The medial wall may be part of the bladder.*

vi. Closure of the canal is affected by approximating the inguinal ligament to the pectineal fascia, or Pectineal Ligament.

vii. The index finger of the left hand protects the femoral vein during the insertion of the sutures.

viii. The wound is closed.

Femoral Hernia Repair – Abdominal Approach
(Cheatle, Henry and McEvedy)

i. An incision is made over the lateral aspect of the rectus sheath (McEvedy), midline, paramedian or transverse (Cheatle and Henry).

ii. It is deepened through the anterior abdominal wall to expose the peritoneum.

iii. The peritoneum is followed down to the neck of the sac and the procedure is as described for the other approaches.

iv. If difficulty is encountered, another incision is made directly over the hernia; however, with the McEvedy approach a downward extension of the incision gives direct access to the hernia.

v. The inguinal ligament is sutured to Pectineal Ligament to obliterate the aperture.

vi. The wall of the abdomen is repaired and the wound closed.

43. UMBILICAL HERNIA REPAIR IN CHILDREN

i. The umbilicus is held up and a small transverse incision is made below it so that on replacing the umbilicus it forms its lower margin.

ii. The incision is deepened to the rectus sheath, and the emerging sac separated from the surrounding structures by dissecting around it with a curved scissors or artery forceps.

iii. The overlying fascia is divided and the peritoneum opened.

iv. The peritoneum is repaired separately, and the margins of the defect overlapped, or both layers are overlapped together as in a "Mayo" operation.

v. The skin is approximated with subcuticular catgut sutures.

vi. The area may be covered with a plastic dressing.

44. UMBILICAL HERNIA REPAIR IN THE ADULT
(Mayo)

i. A transverse elliptical incision is made over the mass to include the umbilicus and one-third of the bulge. This skin is subsequently removed with the adherent sac.

ii. The incision is deepened all round to expose the rectus sheath.

iii. The hernia is held with gauze and by sharp dissection over the surface of the sheath, the neck is reached.

iv. The neck of the sac is opened all round, the contents are replaced after division and ligation of adhesions.

v. The defect is repaired by overlapping the fat-free edges and surfaces by means of mattress sutures employing non-absorbable material; lateral extensions into the rectus sheath may facilitate the repair.

vi. The wound is closed.

45. INCISIONAL HERNIA REPAIR
Keel Repair (Maingot)

i. An elliptical incision is made over the hernia.

ii. The incision is deepened to the fibrous tissue layer overlying the defect.

iii. By sharp dissection and keeping on the surface of this layer, the defect is freed from the oval portion of skin. Small openings inadvertently made in the peritoneum are closed with catgut.

iv. The dissection is extended over the rectus sheath and external oblique until a wide mobilisation is achieved.

v. The sac is then inverted and the edges of the defect are brought together with interrupted mattress sutures.

vi. A continuous right-angled Cushing suture is then introduced for further support.

vii. Following meticulous haemostasis and obliteration of dead space, the wound is closed.

Cattell advises opening the sac, repairing the peritoneum at its neck but including all layers of abdominal wall that are fused to the edge of the defect with a continuous locking chromic catgut suture.

A second layer reinforces this repair and includes a small fringe of the sac, deliberately preserved. The remainder of the sac is excised.

46. OPERATIONS FOR UNDESCENDED TESTICLE

i. A transverse skin incision is made and carefully deepened to expose the external oblique and the testicle if it is lying in the superficial inguinal pouch.

ii. The testis is freed from its gubernacular attachments.

iii. The external oblique is opened to expose the cord and the internal ring.

iv. If present, an indirect hernia is dissected free of the cord structures and its neck transfixed and ligated. If the sac extends down to the testis, the distal portion of the sac may be left.

v. The testis is held and the cord mobilised by sharp and blunt dissection (Lahey swabs) well above the internal ring.

vi. A passage to the scrotum is opened digitally.

vii. The thigh and scrotum are now incised and the posterior edges where they readily come into contact united with catgut sutures.

viii. The testis is now anchored by passing a black silk suture through the tunica albuginea brought down through the scrotum and anchored to the fascia lata of the thigh.

ix. The union of scrotum to thigh is now completed anteriorly with interrupted non-absorbable sutures. Alternatively, the testicle may be placed in the subcutaneous pouch of the scrotum and anchored to the thigh with a non-absorbable suture (Bevan).

x. The upper wound is closed.

xi. Three months later, the scrotum and testis are separated from the thigh.

CHAPTER V

GALL BLADDER, BILE DUCTS AND PANCREAS

47 AND 48. CHOLECYSTECTOMY AND CHOLEDOCHOTOMY

General principles

i. An operation that may be extremely difficult. Two assistants are advised.

ii. Vitamin K may be required with recent biliary obstruction.

iii. A vertical right paramedian incision is made for patients who have narrow costal angles or in whom the diagnosis is in doubt. An oblique subcostal incision may be employed if the costal angle is wide. Note that the transversus abdominis may be seen posterior to the divided rectus abdominis.

iv. Open the peritoneum and explore – particularly note hiatus, stomach, duodenum, pancreas and liver. Lift the right hepatic lobe and allow air to pass behind it. Insert the left index finger into the Foramen of Winslow to palpate the bile duct.*

v. Decide on the operation – it may be necessary to preserve the gall-bladder for use as a by-pass.

Cholecystectomy

i. Pack off the lesser curvature of the stomach to the left, the duodenum and colon downwards and insert retractors. A third retractor on the liver exposes the cystic duct area.

ii. To aid dissection apply sponge-holding forceps to the fundus of the gall bladder and Dennis Browne's tonsil forceps (with ratchet) to Hartmann's pouch to manipulate the cystic duct.

iii. Divide and strip off the peritoneum over the ducts. With further dissection identify the cystic artery by tracing it to the gall bladder.
Free and divide it between ligatures.

iv. *Note.* – There may be five structures behind or close to the cystic duct:

(a) The hepatic artery or right hepatic artery.

(b) Cystic vessels may be multiple.

(c) The right hepatic duct.

(d) A right accessory hepatic duct.

(e) Medially the portal vein.

v. Dissect further to show clearly the termination of the cystic duct – ligate. An operative cholangiogram may now be carried out through a catheter introduced into the cystic duct. It may then be divided close to the common bile duct. (The distal cut end may be held by the tip of a Moyniham forcep.)

vi. Remove the gall bladder by dividing its attachments to the liver and its peritoneal reflection. Suture the gall bladder bed *pari passu* with the removal of the gall bladder. A corrugated drain is left draining the gall bladder area and is brought out through a separate opening in the flank.

vii. There are five classical indications for opening the common bile duct if the operation cholangiogram is not used:

(a) If a stone is palpable or fine debris or white bile is found on needle aspiration.

(b) A dilated common bile duct.

(c) A history of obstructive jaundice.

(d) The gall bladder which contains a large number of small stones.

(e) A history of cholangitis. (Charcot's intermittent fever.)

viii. To open the common bile duct free a part of its anterior wall above the duodenum, then two stay sutures are inserted through the wall.

ix. If you doubt the structure that you are dissecting, aspirate the contents with a needle.

x. Prior to opening the common bile duct, pack off the area and have a sucker in readiness.

xi. The stay sutures are held taut and a small longitudinal cut is made in the common bile duct.

xii. The duct is explored. A variety of instruments are available, for example, Bakes dilators, Lister's bougies, gum elastic bougies, Desjardin's forceps, scoops or finger.

xiii. After removal of any stones and debris, the vessel is washed out with saline.

xiv. An attempt is now made to dilate the Sphincter of Oddi by the passage of bougies. These instruments must be passed through the sphincter.

xv. If unsuccessful, the second part of the duodenum is mobilised, opened vertically, and the Sphincter of Oddi is divided under vision; or a choledochogram is taken to verify that all obstructions have been removed.

xvi. Find the site of the sphincteric opening by palpating the tip of a probe passed down the common bile duct from above.

xvii. Divide the sphincter at 12 o'clock, or sphincteroplasty may be carried out.

xviii. Close the duodenum with two layers transversely.

xix. Insert T-tube into supraduodenal common duct opening. Close opening around tube with catgut.

xx. Add a corrugated rubber strip to drain area of gall bladder bed. Place surgical haemostatic gauze into gall bladder bed if oozy.

xxi. Bring out drainage tubes carefully through a separate opening.

Post-operative care

i. If the T-tube is pulled out by accident, open the abdomen and replace it immediately.

ii. Clamp T-tube from fifth day.

iii. Remove the corrugated tube on the fifth day.

iv. Choledochogram is taken on the tenth day.

v. Remove the T-tube if X-ray is satisfactory.

49. CHOLECYSTOSTOMY

How do you treat a gangrenous gall bladder? The general principle is that in the presence of gangrene minimal surgery is carried out.

i. An intravenous drip, and gastric suction are used until resuscitated. Antibiotics are commenced.

ii. Open the abdomen.

iii. Cut away the gangrenous portion after careful "packing". Suck out and remove the contents. Suture a drainage tube into the gall bladder with catgut.

iv. Close the abdomen bringing the tube out through a separate stab wound.

50 CHOLECYSTOJEJUNOSTOMY AND ENTERO-ENTEROSTOMY (Braun)

i. A right vertical incision is made.

ii. Bring up the first jejunal loop across the colon so that it lies without tension.

iii. Aspirate the gall bladder if necessary, then anastomose the small bowel to it with at least two layers of closely inserted sutures. The anastomosis lies about 50 cm from the duodenojejunal flexure.

iv. By-pass this anastomosis below by anastomosing the two limbs of the loop together (side-to-side) with two layers of catgut.

v. Close wound carefully – these patients are usually cachectic and wound dehiscence may occur.

51. EXPLORATION OF PANCREAS FOR ADENOMA

i. A right paramedian incision is made.

ii. Mobilise the greater curvature of stomach, dividing the gastrocolic ligament and any adhesions between stomach and pancreas to visualise and palpate the body of the pancreas with the flat of the hand.

iii. To palpate tail of pancreas, mobilise it with the spleen by dividing the peritoneum lateral to the spleen.

iv. To palpate the head of pancreas, mobilise the duodenum by dividing the peritoneum on its lateral aspect (Kocher). Mobilise the head and the duodenum by blunt dissection and palpate the head between finger and thumb.

52. PARTIAL PANCREATICODUODENECTOMY

i. Remember intravenous drip, Ryle's tube and Vitamin K.

ii. A long right paramedian incision is made.

iii. Open the peritoneum and explore.

iv. Expose the duodenum by mobilising the right half of the transverse colon and its hepatic flexure by dividing its peritoneal reflections.

v. Identify and dissect out the common bile duct above the duodenum.

vi. Mobilise the duodenum by dividing the peritoneum along its right border.

vii. Identify the superior mesenteric vessels carefully, palpate along them, and finally ensure that these vessels and the inferior vena cava are not implicated.

viii. Divide the common bile duct above the duodenum.

ix. Mobilise the pyloric antrum and the first part of the duodenum by dividing the omentum and the right gastric, gastro-duodenal and right gastro-epiploic vessels.

x. Free and divide the distal part of the duodenum or jejunum. Ligate the inferior pancreaticoduodenal vessels.

xi. With great care dissect out the superior mesenteric vessels, tying the short stubby veins.* Carefully divide the neck of the pancreas.

xii. Bring the jejunum up in front of or behind the colon and implant into it from above downwards, the common bile duct, the pancreatic duct (or the cut end of the pancreas), and the stomach.

xiii. Close the abdomen.

53. STRICTURE OF COMMON BILE DUCT

Five general principles at laparotomy

i. At laparotomy check on cause and nature of the biliary obstruction.

ii. There must be no tension at the suture line.

iii. In the anastomosis there must be mucosa to mucosa apposition.*

iv. A loop of Roux "Y" of jejunum is used if the common bile duct cannot be reconstituted.

v. Avoid bringing out the T-tube through the anastomosis.

Operation for Bile Duct Strictures

Remember intravenous drip, Ryle's tube and Vitamin K.

i. A long right paramedian incision, with or without T-extension to right, is made.

ii. Mobilise the hepatic flexure to expose the duodenum.

iii. Mobilise the duodenum by Kocher's manoeuvre, search for the lower end of duct. The duodenum may be opened and a probe passed through Sphincter of Oddi to help.

iv. Employ a needle to identify the upper end, starting close to hilum of the liver.

v. Piecemeal removal of liver at the hilum may help in the discovery of the duct.

vi. The common bile duct lymph gland is helpful to indicate the site of the duct.

vii. Join up the ends of the duct if possible after excising stricture or bring up loop of jejunum. A jejunal mucosal tube may be brought up and approximated to the intra-hepatic ducts within the liver if the extra-hepatic ducts are absent (Rodney Smith). If a loop of jejunum is used, an entero-anastomosis is performed below.

viii. The anastomosis may be made over a tube to help in the identification and suture of the lateral and anterior edges of the anastomosis. A rubber tube can be left in to be passed per rectum later or a Y-shaped vitallium or similar tube can be left in permanently, or drainage may be established through a transhepatic tube. (Rodney Smith.)

ix. The jejunum profitably may be anchored to the liver to avoid "drag".

x. The abdomen is closed with a drain at site of the anastomosis.

CHAPTER VI

LIVER AND SPLEEN

54. Splenectomy
55. Portal Hypertension. The Treatment of Haemorrhage
56. Portocaval Anastomosis
57. Excision of Left Lobe of Liver
58. Oesophageal Transection for Oesophageal Varices
59. Sub-cardiac Porto-azygos Disconnexion
60. Right Hepatic Lobectomy

54. SPLENECTOMY

i. General anaesthesia, an intravenous infusion, and a Ryle's tube are used.

ii. A long left paramedian, or a left oblique subcostal incision is made. Rarely, a thoraco-abdominal incision is required.

iii. The abdomen is opened and explored; spleniculi are sought if relevant.

iv. The spleen is drawn to the right with the left hand and mobilised by dividing the adhesions on its lateral aspect, the left leaf of the lieno-renal ligament and the attachments to the splenic flexure.

v. The tail of the pancreas and the spleen can be brought into the wound by blunt dissection behind the pancreas.

vi. The gastrosplenic ligament and its vessels are divided to expose the tail of the pancreas and the splenic vessels.

vii. The main vessels are doubly ligated close to the spleen to avoid pancreatic damage, and individually ligated to avoid the development of arteriovenous fistulae.

viii. The raw area of the splenic bed is checked for bleeding and the tail of the pancreas is allowed to fall back.

ix. The abdomen is carefully closed with non-absorbable sutures to avoid wound dehiscence upon the release of pancreatic ferments.

55. PORTAL HYPERTENSION

Fresh blood is used to make up platelets and other clotting factors. Vitamin K1 10 mg is administered intramuscularly daily. To remove blood from bowel, purge with Mag. Sulphate orally and employ enemata.

Treatments for Haemorrhage

Medical management

i. Vasopressin 20 units in 100 ml of 5 per cent dextrose intravenously administered over 20 minutes, repeated after four hours. It induces splanchnic arteriolar vasoconstriction.

ii. Gastric hypothermia may be tried by circulating ethanol-water mixture at 0°C through intragastric balloon (1–3 days).

iii. Oesophageal tamponage, maximum use 36 hours. Aspirate pharynx.

Pre-operative care

i. The patient is on a low protein diet 20 g per day, starting four days before operation.

ii. A course of Neomycin is started two days before operation.

Surgical treatment

i. Portocaval anastomosis.

ii. Lienorenal anastomosis.

iii. Gastric or oesophageal transection.

iv. High proximal gastrectomy.

Normal portal vein pressure is 15 cm of saline, more than double this pressure is abnormal.

56. PORTOCAVAL ANASTOMOSIS

i. Controlled respiration anaesthesia, intravenous drip, diathermy, and water manometer filled with potassium citrate are used.

ii. The patient lies supine and tilted to the left supported by a sandbag behind the right shoulder and buttock.

iii. A thoraco-abdominal approach is made by excising the right ninth rib subperiosteally and dividing the costal margin and the anterior abdominal wall muscles in line with the incision.

iv. The pleura and peritoneum are opened. The diaphragm is divided down to its central tendon.

v. A self-retaining retractor is inserted. The portal pressure is recorded.

vi. The hepatic flexure is freed to expose the duodenum.

vii. The operation field is packed off.

viii. The peritoneum overlying the free edge of the lesser omentum, second part of duodenum, and lateral aspect of the vena cava is divided.

ix. The portal vein, its tributaries, and the inferior vena cava are dissected out and encircled with sutures.

x. A Blalock clamp is placed down on the portal vein, the portal vein above the clamp is tied and divided.

xi. The inferior vena cava is partially clamped and a vertical opening the size of the cut end of the portal vein made in it.

xii. Employing a fine arterial suture an end-to-side anastomosis is made using everting mattress sutures.

xiii. The clamps are removed and haemostasis obtained. A liver biopsy may be taken.

xiv. The diaphragm and costal cartilage are reconstituted.

xv. The lung is inflated in all parts and the chest closed with an under-water seal.

57. EXCISION OF LEFT LOBE OF LIVER

i. A Ryle's tube, intravenous drip, and diathermy are used. Vitamin K may be necessary.

ii. A long left paramedian incision is made.

iii. The abdomen is opened and explored.

iv. The falciform ligament and the ligamentum teres are divided.

v. The left lobe is drawn to the right and mobilised by dividing the triangular ligament and the upper part of the lesser omentum.

vi. The inferior vena cava is sought.

vii. The peritoneum overlying the bile ducts is now divided to expose the branches.

viii. The left hepatic duct, the left hepatic artery and the left branch of the portal vein are ligated and divided.

ix. The left lobe is now excised carefully with diathermy and its left hepatic vein ligated and divided. The line of division is made from above downwards from the attachment line of the falciform ligament in front and the left side of the fissure of the ductus venosus and transverse fissure behind.

x. The falciform ligament may be used to cover the raw area of the liver.

xi. The wound is closed and drained.

58. OESOPHAGEAL TRANSECTION FOR OESOPHAGEAL VARICES

i. Anaesthesia using a double-lumen tube, diathermy and intravenous drip are required. The patient lies in the lateral position on his right side.

ii. The chest is opened through the bed of the eighth rib.

iii. The pleura is opened and a self-retaining retractor inserted.

iv. The lower lobe of the lung is mobilised by dividing the pulmonary ligament to expose the mediastinal pleura covering the oesophagus.

v. The mediastinal pleura is picked up and divided to expose the oesophagus.

vi. The oesophagus is mobilised and its lower end clamped.

vii. The oesophagus is divided vertically for 5 cm to expose the mucosa.

viii. The mucosa is mobilised circumferentially. The submucous vessels are under-run.

ix. The mucosa is divided transversely and resutured to complete division of the veins.

x. The clamp is removed and a check for haemorrhage is made.

xi. The muscle layer of the oesophagus and the mediastinal pleura are re-united.

xii. The lung is inflated.

xiii. The chest is closed with under-water seal.

59. SUB-CARDIAC PORTO-AZYGOS DISCONNEXION (Tanner)

i. Controlled respiration anaesthesia, intravenous drip, and diathermy are required.

ii. Abdominothoracic approach through the bed of the left ninth rib provides easy access.

iii. The diaphragm is divided down to the oesophagus.

iv. The lower part of the oesophagus (6 cm) and the upper part of the stomach (8 cm) are freed.

v. The stomach is divided 5 cm below the oesophagus.

vi. The stomach is reconstituted by re-anastomosis with two layers of catgut.

vii. Tanner recommends closing the lesser curve part of the lower incision and anastomosing the upper end to the outer two-thirds of the lower end. The upper segment is overlapped by the lower segment as an added precaution.

viii. Pyloroplasty or gastrojejunostomy is performed because the vagal nerves have been divided.*

ix. The lung is inflated. An underwater seal chest drain is inserted. The diaphragm and wound are closed.

60. RIGHT HEPATIC LOBECTOMY

i. The patient lies supine with a sandbag placed under the right shoulder and buttock. Tilting the table helps the various procedures.

ii. The abdomen is opened through a right paramedian incision and explored. If operable this approach is converted into a thoraco-abdominal incision using the seventh or eighth rib-beds and dividing the costal cartilage.

iii. The lung is collapsed and packed off to expose the inferior vena cava (and a self-retaining retractor is introduced.) The diaphragm is divided down to the vein and a tape is placed loosely around the inferior vena cava to establish control if the need should arise.

iv. At the portahepatis the cystic duct and artery, then the right hepatic duct, artery and right branch of portal vein are doubly ligated and divided.

v. The ligamentum teres is sectioned and a clamp is left on its hepatic side to act as a retractor.

vi. The duodenum and head of pancreas are mobilised to demonstrate the inferior vena cava, a tape is placed around the vein above the renal veins.

vii. The right lobe is mobilised dividing the right triangular and posterior layers of the coronary ligament together with small hepatic veins draining into the inferior vena cava to reach the level of the main hepatic veins.

viii. The liver is drawn to the left. The tongue of liver passing behind the right edge of the inferior vena cava is freed to reveal the inferior border of the right hepatic vein.

ix. The right hepatic vein is separated from the left hepatic vein with artery forceps introduced from below upwards ligated and divided.

x. The liver is allowed to fall back and the gall-bladder is dissected to the right to reveal the line of section of the liver which runs from the left border of the gall-bladder bed to the vena cava.

xi. The liver may be divided with a fine artery forceps that allows identification of vessels and ducts. Mattress sutures may be employed to control venous oozing. The right lobe is removed.

xii. The cut surface of the left lobe may be covered with the falciform ligament.

xiii. A T-tube is placed in the common bile duct and a corrugated drain below the right diaphragm.

xiv. The chest wound and diaphragm are closed and the chest drained with an underwater seal drain.

xv. Vitamin K is administered for the following eight days.

CHAPTER VII

NECK AND SALIVARY GLANDS

61. TRACHEOSTOMY

i. The head is extended and held in the sagittal plane; a sandbag is placed between the shoulders. A conscious child is best wrapped in a blanket and its head held steady by an assistant.

ii. General, local or no anaesthesia is used, depending on circumstances.

iii. A vertical incision is made below the thyroid cartilage (down to the sternum in children). Grip the thyroid cartilage with thumb and forefinger of the left hand.*

iv. Deepen the incision, divide the deep fascia, and separate the sternohyoid and sternothyroid muscles.

v. Ligate the transverse branches of the anterior jugular veins.

vi. Identify the thyroid isthmus, mobilise and divide it between haemostats.

vii. Five per cent cocaine may be injected into the trachea to stop coughing.

viii. Divide the tracheal ring (third or fourth) with knife edge uppermost holding the cricoid steady with a hook.* Excise the edges of the opening if possible to facilitate insertion of the tube. Cover the opening with a swab to avoid contaminations due to explosive cough.

ix. Hold the trachea open with a tracheal dilator and insert the tube. The trachea or a turned-back flap of it may be sutured to the skin.

x. The wound is closed with one or two interrupted skin sutures.

xi. The tube is held in position with tapes tied around the neck.

Five dangers in front of the trachea in children

i. Innominate vein.

ii. Anterior jugular veins.

iii. Thyroid isthmus or thymus.

iv. Inferior thyroid vein.

v. Arteria thyroidea ima.

Postoperative phase (requires special nursing care)

i. At the bedside a spare tube and introducer, a suction apparatus and fine catheter are available.

ii. Remove and clean inner tube every four hours.

iii. Humidifier or mucolytic aerosols are useful for thinning viscid secretions.

iv. Remove tube finally in theatre. A tracheostomy set is available should the need arise.

v. If the trachea collapses, suture its wall to the skin.

62. LARYNGOSTOMY

Laryngostomy: Opening the cricothyroid space. It is impracticable in children as the space is too small.

i. Local anaesthesia is used.

ii. The neck is fully extended.

iii. A transverse cut is made above the cricoid.

iv. The incision is deepened and the cricothyroid membrane is divided.

v. The laryngostomy tube is inserted.

63. LARYNGOFISSURE AND THYROTOMY

i. General anaesthesia is used, or local and cocaine.

ii. Tilt the table to avoid blood descending to the lungs, or tilt the head only.

iii. A mid-line incision is made from the hyoid to the suprasternal notch.

iv. Divide the deep fascia and isthmus of the thyroid gland.

v. Perform a tracheostomy and put in tube and connect the anaesthetic machine to it.

vi. Expose the cricothyroid membrane and remove the cricothyroid gland if present.

vii. Divide the perichondrium and thyroid cartilage on the side opposite the growth.

viii. Open the larynx and pack off.

ix. Excise cartilage on the affected side with the growth on the cord, the false cord above and subglottic healthy tissue below. Suture together the divided perichondrium of the thyroid cartilage.

x. Repair the deep fascia down to the tracheostomy tube.

xi. The tracheostomy is left for forty-eight hours.

xii. Sit the patient up after the operation. Feed through a stomach tube if difficulty with swallowing is encountered, e.g. if the arytenoid cartilages have been removed.

64. LARYNGECTOMY

i. General anaesthesia is employed through an endotracheal tube or through a tracheostomy. An oesophageal tube is *in situ.*

ii. A U-shaped incision is used.

iii. The thyroid isthmus is divided and the gland separated to expose the upper part of the trachea. The superior thyroid vessels are divided and ligated.

iv. The thyroid cartilage is freed of its muscular and fibrous attachments including the sternothyroid, thyrohyoid, inferior constrictor, lateral thyrohyoid ligament and stylopharyngeus.

v. The thyrohyoid membrane is divided, thus opening the larynx.

vi. The pharyngeal mucosa is divided above the thyroid cartilage and extended round the aryepiglottic folds and the arytenoid processes. The attachment of the epiglottis to the hyoid is severed. The pharynx is packed off.

vii. The larynx now freed is dissected forwards off the oesophagus.

viii. The trachea is divided below the cricoid cartilage and the larynx removed.

ix. The opening in the pharynx is closed, using the submucosa and muscle layers resulting in a T-shaped closure.

x. The muscles and deep fascia are united in mid-line.

xi. The lower end of the trachea is brought out of the wound and its edges sutured to the skin.

xii. The wound is closed.

65. EXCISION OF THYROGLOSSAL FISTULA

i. Endotracheal anaesthesia is used. The neck is extended by placing a sandbag between the shoulders.

ii. Methylene blue is injected into the fistula.

iii. A transverse skin incision is made to include the fistulous opening.

iv. The tract is dissected upwards and removed with the central portion of the hyoid bone to which it is intimately connected (Sistrunk). The dissection is continued upwards, and the remaining part of the fistula is removed. An assistant inserting a finger into the mouth and pushing down the foramen caecum may facilitate the dissection.

66. EXCISION OF BRANCHIAL FISTULA

i. General anaesthesia is used. The head is turned to the opposite side.

ii. The fistula is injected with methylene blue to aid dissection.

iii. A second skin crease incision placed at a higher level aids the mobilisation.

iv. The track passes between the internal and external carotids and the hypoglossal and glossopharyngeal nerves.

v. It is traced to the pharyngeal wall and tied off, or it may be invaginated into the pharynx and then tied off.

67. EXCISION OF SUBMANDIBULAR GLAND

i. A curved skin crease incision is made over the gland, the posterior part of the incision lies one fingerbreadth below the angle of the jaw to avoid the cervical branch of the facial nerve. The incision is deepened through the platysma and the flaps reflected.

ii. The facial vessels are ligated and divided above as they cross the mandible.

iii. The upper border of the gland is freed.

iv. The common facial vein is exposed behind the gland, ligated and divided.

v. The anterior margin of the sternomastoid is mobilised and the facial artery arising from the external carotid is identified, ligated and divided. The hypoglossal nerve is seen and preserved.

vi. The superficial part of the gland is mobilised anteriorly by raising it from the mylohyoid muscle.

vii. The deep part of the gland and its duct is freed from the hyoglossus muscle. The lingual nerve is seen above and is preserved.

viii. The deep part is freed and the duct divided.

68. EXCISION OF TUBERCULOUS GLANDS OF NECK

For a localised mass in the neck

i. Antibiotic cover is used to avoid the danger of miliary spread.

ii. Endotracheal anaesthesia is employed.

iii. A crease incision is made either across the mass or just above.

iv. The incision is deepened to expose the sternomastoid and its anterior border.

v. The deep fascia is divided and the gland surface reached.

vi. Once on the glands "stick close to them".

vii. Raise by blunt dissection the various periglandular adhesions, examine them and tie them if necessary.

viii. The common facial vein and tributaries require division. Identify the carotid sheath and its contents.

ix. The spinal accessory nerve crosses the palpable transverse process of the atlas and is more superficial in the posterior triangle, therefore it is more easily damaged in that area.

x. The great auricular nerve may be damaged and lead to an area of paraesthesia in front of the angle of the jaw.

xi. If an abscess is pointing through the skin, it may be drained below the wound for 48 hours.

xii. The affected glands are removed and the platysma and skin are closed.

69. COMPLETE UNILATERAL BLOCK DISSECTION OF NECK

The object is to remove a block of tissue containing lymphatic glands and lymphatics extending from the lower border of the mandible (with or without the tail of the parotid) to the mastoid; limited posteriorly by the anterior border of Trapezius; by the clavicle and the opposite side of the midline of the neck.

i. Endotracheal anaesthesia is employed, a sandbag is placed between the shoulders and the head turned to the opposite side.

ii. The incision commences behind the mastoid process, curves downwards and forwards 3 cm below the angle of the jaw, and then upwards to terminate on the chin just the other side* of the mid-line. A vertical incision is made from the middle of this incision down to the middle of the clavicle.

iii. The skin flaps are reflected back.

iv. Two veins are divided, one in front of and one behind the sternomastoid. Divide the sternomastoid just above the clavicle, dividing the external jugular vein posteriorly. Dissect out the internal jugular vein anteriorly from the carotid sheath and divide it. It is dangerous to divide the internal jugular vein if it has been resected on the opposite side.

v. **Clearance of supraclavicular fossa and division of omohyoid**
Divide along the clavicle, the deep fascia, omohyoid fascia and muscle until the prevertebral fascia is reached. The brachial nerves are seen covered by a thin layer of prevertebral fascia. Branches of the subclavian vessels are ligated. The dissection reaches the anterior border of the Trapezius. The thoracic duct on the left side is preserved.

vi. **Continuation of dissection to hyoid level**
The block of tissue containing the internal jugular vein is dissected up until the level of the hyoid is reached. The tributaries of the internal jugular, middle and superior thyroid and later on the common facial veins are divided.

vii. **The digastric landmark**
This white shining structure is identified below the submandibular gland and above the level of the hyoid. Identify the hypoglossal nerve, then divide the central tendon of the digastric muscle to open up the dissection. At this stage the common facial vein is divided.

viii. Identify the facial and occipital arteries arising from external carotid, and divide them between ligatures.

ix. **Dissection of submental triangle**
Continue the dissection upwards over the mylohyoid (to the lower border of the jaw), raising the submandibular gland.

x. **Dislocation of submandibular gland**
Dissect out the gland including its deep portion, divide the duct close to the gland and turn it upwards.

xi. **Ligation of internal jugular vein**
Dissect out this enlarging structure carefully and doubly ligate and divide it at the base of the skull.

xii. **Division of mass**
Commencing posteriorly divide the sternomastoid and digastric, remove the tail of parotid if necessary, then cut along the lower border of jaw, ligating the facial vessels, until the opposite side of the midline is reached and the mass removed.

xiii. Close the skin and drain the wound.

70. SUB-TOTAL THYROIDECTOMY

i. Endotracheal anaesthesia is essential.

ii. Place a sandbag between the shoulders to extend the neck.

iii. A collar incision is made one finger-breadth above the sternal notch.

iv. Deepen the incision through the platysma on both sides of the neck to expose the deep fascia.

v. By sharp dissection raise the upper flap until the thyroid notch is reached and the lower flap down to the suprasternal notch.

vi. Joll's self-retaining retractor is then introduced and skin towels applied.

vii. Divide the deep fascia vertically in the midline until the veins on the thyroid isthmus are exposed.

viii. Raise the strap muscles on one side to expose the lateral lobe, insert retractors and continue the dissection until the entire lobe is clearly visible. Note the deep layer of strap muscle is closely adherent to the gland.

ix. Divide and ligate the middle thyroid vein.

x. Dislocate the lateral lobe into wound. If necessary, to improve exposure, divide strap muscles between forceps at level of the cricoid cartilage, to preserve their nerve supply.

xi. Dissect laterally and posteriorly to the lobe of the thyroid and identify inferior thyroid artery, recurrent laryngeal nerve and parathyroids. Ligate the artery in continuity. Note that some surgeons do not attempt to find the recurrent nerves, but in this case dissect out the artery and ligate it well away from the gland.

xii. Mobilise the upper pole away from the pharynx; insert Kocher's director behind it and doubly ligate superior thyroid vessels. Apply artery forceps to the upper pole beyond the ligatures and by dividing the intervening tissues, the upper pole is freed.

xiii. Expose the front of the trachea by dividing inferior thyroid veins and if present, free the pyramidal lobe.

xiv. Change to the opposite side of the patient and free the other lobe and deal similarly with its vessels.

xv. Apply a ring of forceps around the gland on the visible vessels and divide the gland. Continue by applying forceps to gland substance until the trachea is reached. Most of the lateral lobes, the whole of the isthmus and pyramidal lobe are removed. Two small posterior portions of gland are left on either side of the trachea. One-eighth of the gland is conserved.

xvi. Suture the remaining part of the gland if it is bleeding to the side of the trachea.

xvii. Insert two drains emerging through the deep fascia at the lateral aspects of the wound.

xviii. Close the deep fascia.

xix. Remove sandbag from beneath shoulders and approximate platysma with fine catgut.

xx. Suture drainage tubes to the skin.

xxi. Close the wound with clips.

Five important points

i. If in difficulties, search for and identify trachea.

ii. The inferior thyroid arteries are found lateral to the gland. They are usually found deep to an opaque fascia lateral to the lateral lobes of the gland, and emerging from beneath the carotid sheath.

iii. Beware of air-embolism, and prevent oozing of blood during the entire procedure.

iv. Divide the strap muscles immediately any technical difficulty is encountered.

v. When an area oozes unduly, pack it off carefully and do some other part of the dissection and return to it later.

71. EXCISION AND REPAIR OF PHARYNGEAL POUCH

i. General anaesthesia is used. A large oesophageal tube may be guided into the oesophagus below the pouch during the operation. It helps to identify the neck of the sac.

ii. An incision is made along the anterior border of the left sterno-mastoid.

iii. The pouch neck lies at the level of the cricoid.

iv. Deepen the incision to expose the left lobe of the thyroid gland and the carotid sheath. The pouch lies between them.

v. To improve access, divide the omohyoid muscle.

vi. Retract the carotid sheath laterally.

vii. Divide the middle thyroid vein and the superior thyroid vessels, and retract the thyroid lobe medially.

viii. The oesophageal tube is passed down into the oesophagus.

ix. Dissect the sac to its neck and divide its fascial covering, leaving a 1 cm fringe for closure.

x. Excise the sac and close the mucosa.

xi. Close the thinned-out fibromuscular fringe over it, establishing a second layer.

xii. Repair the deep fascia.

xiii. Drain the wound.

72. SUPERFICIAL PAROTIDECTOMY

i. General anaesthesia. Warn the patient of possible damage to the facial nerve, or even its deliberate removal if found necessary. Hypotensive agents are helpful to reduce haemorrhage.

ii. Infiltrate the area with dilute adrenalin solution (1:150,000).

iii. The incision runs vertically down just in front of the pinna, curves backwards below it, then extends forwards in a skin crease across the neck.

iv. The skin flaps are widely mobilised and held back by stay sutures to reveal all aspects of the gland. The great auricular nerve may be preserved or sacrificed.

v. There are five approaches to the facial nerve and its branches:

(a) From in front of the gland, tracing back any branch or branches of the nerve.

(b) From behind the gland, identifying the bony meatus and following up the posterior belly of the digastric.

(c) Following up the posterior facial vein; the nerve crosses in front of it.

(d) Removing the mastoid process.

(e) Tracing back in particular the cervical branch of the nerve.

vi. A combination of these methods is useful if much bleeding is encountered. The bleeding area is packed, and one of the alternative dissections followed in the meantime.

vii. A nerve stimulator is sometimes useful.

viii. A frozen section should be obtained if diagnosis is doubtful.

ix. The superficial lobe is removed, preserving the facial nerve.

73. TOTAL PAROTIDECTOMY FOR CARCINOMA

i. Make sure the patient is aware that facial paralysis will occur.

ii. Endotracheal anaesthesia is used.

iii. A vertical incision is made, commencing at the zygoma, in front of the pinna, curving backwards under the lobe of the ear, then forwards across the neck in a skin crease.

iv. The skin flaps are raised to expose all aspects of the gland and the sternomastoid.

v. The posterior facial, the common facial vein and the great auricular nerve are divided.

vi. The deep fascia is divided in front of the sternomastoid to expose the posterior belly of the digastric muscle and its white tendon, the hypoglossal nerve, the stylohyoid muscle and the external carotid artery.

vii. The external carotid is ligated.

viii. Mobilise the anterior margin of the gland by dividing the parotid duct, the facial nerve branches and the transverse facial vessels.

ix. Free the superior aspect by dividing its fascial attachments and the superficial temporal vessels.

x. Dissect posteriorly and divide the facial nerve, the posterior auricular vessels and attachments to the styloid and mastoid processes.

xi. Remove the deep portion together with the posterior part of the ramus of the mandible. A Gigli saw is passed from the angle of the jaw through the sigmoid notch, and the bone is divided. The inferior dental nerve is avoided and preserved.

xii. The maxillary artery is divided and ligated.

xiii. The head of the mandible is freed from the joint.

xiv. The gland and bone are freed from, or removed with, the involved sternomastoid.

xv. Haemostasis is obtained and the wound closed with drainage.

74. EXCISION OF CAROTID BODY TUMOUR

Fifteen to 20 per cent of these tumours are malignant (Lahey and Warren), necessitating excision of the carotid bifurcation. If the internal carotid artery is ligated hemiplegia or death occurs in approximately 25 to 50 per cent of patients.

To avoid this danger the continuity between the common and internal carotid vessels is restored using an autograft, homograft or plastic vessel graft.

CHAPTER VIII

FACE, MOUTH AND JAW

75. Caldwell-Luc Operation
76. Excision of Condyle of Jaw
77. Excision of Mandible
78. Excision of Maxilla
79. Hare-lip and Cleft Palate

75. CALDWELL-LUC OPERATION

i. General anaesthesia with an intra-oral endotracheal tube is employed. The pharynx is packed off. The head-end of the table is raised.

ii. To expose the gingivolabial sulcus the cheek is retracted, and an incision is made through it, extending from the first molar to the lateral incisor tooth.

iii. The periosteum is incised over the canine fossa and elevated upwards, but not as far as the infra-orbital nerve.

iv. Part of the anterior wall of the antrum is removed with gouge and mallet, and the cavity explored.

v. The mucosa of the antrum, if diseased, is excised.

vi. The bony medial wall below the inferior turbinate is removed to allow free drainage of the cavity into the nose.

vii. The mucosa of the sulcus may be repaired, or the antral cavity allowed to drain through it. A pack may be left in if necessary for a few hours.

76. EXCISION OF THE CONDYLE OF THE JAW

i. A vertical incision is made commencing at the lower margin of the zygoma, over the joint and in front of the pulsations of the superficial temporal artery.
A horizontal extension forwards, following the lower border of the zygoma, may be made. The skin flap is reflected.

ii. The neck of the mandible is cleared and divided, preserving the transverse facial vessels, facial nerve branches and the parotid.

iii. The condyle is then freed of the attachments, and excised.

iv. Fat and fascia may be sewn into the gap to avoid ankylosis.

77. EXCISION OF MANDIBLE

i. The patient lies supine with the head turned towards the opposite side. Endotracheal anaesthesia is employed, the pharynx is packed off. The head of the table may be raised to reduce venous congestion.

ii. The tongue is held on a stay suture.

iii. The incision commencing below the lip splits the chin and follows the inferior aspect of the body and posterior aspect of the ascending ramus. For excision of only a segment of the jaw the lip and chin may be divided vertically, after which the skin incision follows the crease lines of the neck.

iv. Deepen the incision to expose, ligate and divide the facial vessels as they cross the jaw.

v. The external surface of the body of the mandible is cleared of the buccinator and masseter.

vi. The mucosa of the gingivolabial sulcus is divided.

vii. A lateral incisor tooth is extracted and the jaw divided with a Gigli saw leaving the symphysis with its attachment of the geniohyoid and genioglossus muscles.

viii. The body of the mandible can now be moved and allows the division or reflexion of mylohyoid and the medial pterygoid muscle.

ix. The inferior dental vessels and nerve are divided.

x. The jaw is rotated to view the coronoid process and the temporal muscle is divided.

xi. The lateral pterygoid is divided.

xii. By dividing the capsule, the condyle of the mandible is now exposed and freed; care is taken to avoid the maxillary artery.

xiii. The ligaments (Stylomandibular, sphenomandibular) are divided and the bone removed.

xiv. Mucosal cover within the mouth is attempted as far as possible.

xv. The skin is closed and the wound drained posteriorly.

xvi. The pharyngeal pack is removed.

xvii. The suture on the tongue may be held in a haemostat and left until consciousness returns.

78. EXCISION OF MAXILLA

i. Obtain the patient's permission to excise the eye if necessary.

ii. General anaesthesia; pack off the pharynx and commence by ligating the external carotid artery (q.v.).

iii. To expose the maxilla the cheek and lip is raised as a flap.

iv. The incision commences below the inner canthus of the eye, skirts the nose and its ala nasi, and divides the upper lip in midline. Transversely it crosses and divides the lower eyelid lateral to the lacrymal punctum, divides the conjunctiva in the lower fornix and ends by crossing the zygoma.

v. The cheek flap is raised and the mucosa of the gingivolabial sulcus divided.

vi. The nasal cartilage is separated from the nasal bone.

vii. The periosteum along the lower edge of the orbit is divided, raised and retracted upwards to expose the orbital floor.

viii. The nasal bone and the nasal process of the maxilla are divided.

ix. A Gigli saw may be introduced through the inferior orbital fissure and brought out medial to the zygomatic prominence. The intervening structures are divided.

x. The central incisor tooth on the affected side is removed. The periosteum of the hard palate is divided. The soft palate is freed. The alveolar and palatal processes of the maxilla are divided with a keyhole saw.

xi. The maxilla is elevated off the pterygoid plates – *not* crushed with lion forceps.

xii. The cheek flap is replaced and sutured.

xiii. A pack is left in the cavity with its end emerging through the mouth.

xiv. The pharyngeal pack is removed.

xv. An obturator is subsequently fitted to fill in the cavity.

79. HARE-LIP AND CLEFT PALATE

i. Classification: Hare-lip may be partial or complete, unilateral or bilateral, with or without cleft palate.

ii. The lip defect is corrected when the infant is feeding well and gaining weight. Repair the palate before speech commences.

iii. Endotracheal anaesthesia is used; the pharynx is packed off.

iv. General principles only are described. The repair of the lip first will exert pressure on the alveolar cleft, tending to close it. At the same time, the flattening of the nose is corrected; the walls of the nasal vestibule are drawn together by excising skin. Ensure that the alar cartilages of the nose are at the same level, and correct the columella length.

v. The lip is repaired in three layers with extensive mobilisation of the orbicularis oris muscle, using a "Z" incision.
By extensive mobilisation, tension is avoided at the suture line. A papilla is left on the lip to allow for linear contraction of the scar.

vi. With the palate, the nasopharyngeal sphincter is reconstituted by some form of pharyngoplasty. The palate is displaced backwards and united, "V-Y" advancement flap or the "four-flap" method may be employed. The hamulus and posterior palatine vessels are divided. The nasal mucoperiosteum requires mobilisation.

vii. Feeding is encouraged immediately after operation.

CHAPTER IX

THORAX

80. BRONCHOSCOPY

Diagnostic or therapeutic, e.g. for removal of foreign bodies or retained sputum. Check for the following problems:

(a) Teeth – septic, loose or porcelain capped.

(b) Full stomach.

(c) Deformed spine.

(d) Large intra-thoracic goitre.

(e) Aneurysm of aorta.

i. Efficient sucker etc., and if necessary biopsy and/or grasping forceps are available.

ii. For diagnostic purposes or removal of foreign body, preferably use intravenous anaesthesia with short acting relaxant and intermittent oxygen insufflation.

iii. For sputum retention use local or no anaesthesia according to condition of patient. Local anaesthesia 4 per cent Xylocaine is applied by repeated pharyngeal spray during inspiration or directly by pledglets held against pharyngeal walls and root of tongue using Krause's forceps.

iv. Patient lies supine, neck flexed forwards, head extended.

v. The bronchoscope may be introduced directly via a laryngoscope.

vi. A gauze swab is placed over the upper teeth, and the fingers of the left hand within the mouth act as a fulcrum and protect the teeth and gums.

vii. The tip of the epiglottis is seen and lifted forwards to view the glottis.

viii. The cords are examined and the instrument is passed through them on inspiration.

ix. The bronchoscope is passed downwards and the carina and bronchi examined. By moving the patient's head, the bronchi may be entered in turn.

In diagnosis, a fibre-optic bronchoscope may be used alone or passed through the rigid bronchoscope. Its manoeuvrable tip may reach more distal and otherwise inaccessible bronchial subdivisions for brush biopsy or forceps biopsy under direct vision.

81. MEDIASTINOSCOPY

i. General anaesthesia is used. The neck is extended. The table is tilted downwards at the foot end by 20° to reduce venous congestion.

ii. A 3 cm incision is drawn transversely 4 cm above the suprasternal notch.

iii. The strap muscles are separated by dividing the midline raphe. Superficial veins are divided if present in the line of access.

iv. The thyroid isthmus is dissected free from the trachea divided and ligated to expose it.

v. The anterior aspect of the trachea is cleared of pretracheal fascia and veins to allow the introduction of the right index finger. The left innominate vein and the innominate artery lie anterior to the finger.

vi. Glands especially if enlarged may be found on either side of the trachea.

vii. The finger may be replaced by a mediastinoscope for further inspection or biopsy of glands under direct vision.

viii. Rarely severe haemorrhage may occur and will require packing and possibly an exploration through a right thoracotomy.

82. INTERCOSTAL DRAINAGE OF EMPYEMA

i. Local anaesthesia is used. P.A. and lateral X-rays are displayed to ascertain site of empyema.

ii. The patient sits up with his arms supported on a bed-table.

iii. Confirm the site by needle aspiration. The intercostal space above the lowest part of the empyema is defined.

iv. Infiltrate local anaesthetic through all the layers of the chest wall at this level.

v. Make an incision through the skin only just large enough to admit a trocar and cannula.

vi. Remove the trocar and cover the open cannula with the thumb.

vii. Pass through a "Whistle-tip" or Argyle catheter.

viii. Remove the cannula, holding the tube.

ix. Fix the tube securely with a stitch or strapping.

x. Connect the tube to an underwater seal.

83. RIB RESECTION FOR EMPYEMA

i. General anaesthesia is used. If a bronchial fistula is present, employ a double-lumen endotracheal tube.

ii. P.A. and lateral X-rays are displayed, preferably with Lipiodol studies.

iii. The patient lies in the lateral position.

iv. Confirm the suitability of the selected rib by needle aspiration of the underlying empyema.

v. Make a 7 cm incision in the line of the rib, starting usually a hands-breadth from the vertebral spines.

vi. Deepen the incision to expose the periosteum, which is then divided along the rib and elevated to expose rib borders.

vii. Use a rougine or Doyen's raspatory to free the rib of periosteum and remove 3 cm of rib with a costotome.

viii. Ligate the intercostal bundle at each end of the rib bed.

ix. Open into the cavity by excising 2 cm^2 of thickened pleura, which is sent for biopsy.

x. Suck out the cavity and break down any loculi with the finger. Retain some pus for culture.

xi. Insert a wide bore tube and close the muscles and skin around it with interrupted sutures.

xii. Secure the tube with a safety-pin passed through its wall and anchor the pin to the skin with strapping.

84. THORACOPLASTY

i. General anaesthesia is employed.

ii. The patient lies on his sound side with the arm held forwards on a Carter-Braine rest.

iii. Approaching the ribs posteriorly, a J-shaped periscapular incision is made, commencing 2·5 cm from the midline and 5 cm below the upper border of the trapezius and terminating below the inferior angle of the scapula on the posterior axillary line.

iv. The posterior aspects of the ribs are exposed by dividing the muscles attached to the scapula mobilising and retracting it.

v. The exposure is then improved by elevating the scapula.

vi. The upper ribs are freed of the scaleni, serratus anterior and serratus posterior superior muscles.

vii. To remove any ribs, the periosteum must be divided and reflected. Posteriorly the costotransverse ligament and the neck of the rib is divided. Anteriorly the rib is divided and the freed segment removed.

viii. In a thoracoplasty, the first rib is freed of periosteum, divided and removed similarly. Great care is taken of the vascular and nerve relations. The second rib and most of the third rib are removed in the first-stage operation, which facilitates similar removal of the first rib.

ix. The upper intercostal bundles are divided.

x. Apicolysis is performed.

xi. The wound is closed.

xii. Further ribs are removed later in successive operations to complete the thoracoplasty.

85. OPEN HEART SURGERY

Principle: Temporarily to exclude heart and lungs from the circulation so that the heart may be emptied and relevant intracardiac procedures be performed under direct vision without undue time limit.

Venous blood is diverted from the heart and by gravity enters a machine where it is oxygenated and returned under pressure to the arterial tree.

Bypass Machines: Numerous types are available comprising an oxygenator, heat exchanger, blood filter and arterial pump, together with suction pump to return spilt blood to the machine.

Oxygenators (usually prepacked and disposable), may be–

i. Rotating discs – exposing blood film to Oxygen/CO2 mixture.

ii. "Bubble" – Oxygen is bubbled through a column of blood which is then filtered to remove bubbles before being returned to the patient.

iii. Membrane – using diffusion of gases through a semipermeable membrane.

Heat exchangers are of the radiator principle, circulating warm or cold water to control temperature of blood passing through them.

Preparation: Pre-operative screening forewarns of:

Septic teeth, infected sputum, coagulation defects, hepatic or renal impairment, Australia antigens.

Procedure:

i. Light general anaesthesia is used.

ii. Monitoring systems are set up and include:
E.C.G.
Central venous pressure line,
Arterial line in radial artery,
Urinary catheter,
Temperature probes – nasopharyngeal, oesophageal, rectal.

iii. With the patient supine a midline incision is made from the suprasternal notch to below xiphisternum.

iv. The sternum is divided in the midline with a power saw and the pericardium opened vertically to expose the heart. Pleurae remain intact.

v. Heparin is administered.

vi. Large cannulae are passed into superior and inferior venae cavae via right atrial appendage and are connected to the machine although kept temporarily clamped.

vii. The ascending aorta is cannulated via a purse-string suture in its wall and the clamped cannula is connected to the machine. Air is excluded.

viii. The clamps are removed and bypass is started.

Additional manoeuvres vary according to the nature of the intracardiac operation and may include:

i. A suction vent in the left ventricle.

ii. Snuggers or snares around the cavae to ensure all blood enters the cannulae and none seeps around them into the right atrium.

iii. Individual cannulation of the coronary orifices via the clamped and opened aortic root.

Closure of Chest

i. After completion of intracardiac procedure the bypass is discontinued and the cannulae removed.

ii. Protamine is given to neutralise the Heparin.

iii. The pericardium is approximated with interrupted sutures when possible.

iv. The sternum is closed with interrupted wire sutures.

v. Pericardial and anterior mediastinal drains are led to underwater drainage and suction.

86. INTRA-CARDIAC PROCEDURES

A complex and rapidly advancing frontier of surgical knowledge and expertise and therefore rapidly changing and soon out of date.

1. Atrial Septal Defects

Secundum. Usually is simple and is closed by direct suture. If combined with partial anomalous venous drainage a patch closure may be necessary to correct it.

Primum. The defect is complex and often involves the mitral valve. It is always closed by a patch graft (pericardium or Dacron) and may involve a valve replacement or valvoplasty.

2. Ventricular Septal Defects

The defect is either in isolation or as part of a complex anomaly. It should always be closed by patch graft either pericardium or Dacron.

There is the danger of imminent heart-block due to the proximity of the conducting bundle at the rim of the defect.

3. Valve Replacements

Homograft, Heterograft, or Prosthetic valve may be used. All have advantages and disadvantages, protagonists and antagonists. All are currently used. All four heart valves may be replaced.

4. Fallot's Tetralogy. Total Correction

i. The relief of the obstruction to outflow tract of right ventricle involves the resection of the hypertrophied muscle, pulmonary valvotomy or valve replacement, with the possible enlargement of outflow tract with pericardial or Dacron gusset.

ii. Closure of ventricular septal defect with pericardial or Dacron patch.

5. Transposition

A complex problem. Blood diversion is possible at level of the atria, ventricles or great vessels.

Mustard's Operation.
Atrial Diversion of Blood.

An inter-atrial baffle of pericardium or Dacron is used to divert pulmonary venous return to right ventricle and caval venous return to left ventricle. Ventricular septal defect must be closed.

Rastelli's Operation.
Ventricular Diversion of Blood.

i. The large ventricular septal defect is so closed to allow the left ventricle to eject through the right ventricular outflow tract into the aorta. The pulmonary artery outlet from the left ventricle is oversewn and closed.

ii. A new outflow for the right ventricle is formed by a Dacron tube with inserted valve, anastomosed between a hole made in the anterior wall of the ventricle and the pulmonary trunk.

Great Vessel Switch.
Diversion of Bood at level of Great Vessels.

The roots of aorta and pulmonary trunk are divided and the vessels "switched" so as to restore normal anatomy. The coronary arteries at the aortic root have until recently been a prohibiting complication. Septal defects must be closed.

6. Coronary Artery Bypass Grafts

i. Localised obstruction in a coronary artery is bypassed using homologous vein anastomosed end-to-side at the root of the aorta and end-to-side to the coronary artery below the obstruction.

ii. The long saphenous or cephalic veins are used.

87. CARDIAC ARREST. EXTERNAL CARDIAC MASSAGE

i. Start external massage immediately.

ii. Put patient supine on a firm surface, clear an airway and use mouth to mouth breathing or administer oxygen via endotracheal tube.

iii. Intermittently, (80 per minute) compress the lower sternum with the flat of the hands laid one above the other.

iv. Institute a stable drip and start administration of 8·4 per cent sodium bicarbonate.

v. On E.C.G. differentiate asystole from ventricular fibrillation. (V.F.).

vi. In V.F. use the electrical defibrillator. Persist at reasonable intervals, continuing external massage between times. Intravenous Lignocaine may subdue persistent ventricular excitability.

vii. In asystole correct any suspected electrolytic imbalance then use calcium chloride 10 per cent and adrenalin 1:10,000 to produce contraction. If V.F. supervenes proceed as in vi above.

88. PNEUMONECTOMY

i. Positive pressure anaesthesia is employed using a double-lumen endotracheal tube.

ii. The lateral or (rarely) prone position may be used.

iii. The chest is opened through the sixth rib bed and any adhesions are divided with scissors. Areas of densely adherent pleura may have to be removed with the lung rather than risk opening a diseased lung.

iv. The perihilar pleura and the pulmonary ligament are divided and reflected to expose the hilum. The pericardium may be opened to help assessment of resectability.

v. The pulmonary veins are dissected and individually ligated and divided. If necessary the left atrial wall may be secured in a vascular clamp and the veins divided flush. The atrial wall is oversewn and the clamp removed.

vi. The adventitial sheath of the pulmonary artery is entered and cleared from the vessel which is then ligated and divided.

vii. The bronchus is clamped distally and divided close to the carina. The open stump which should be short, is closed with interrupted non-absorbable sutures. Alternatively the bronchus may be divided between clamps using a non-crushing one proximally. Sutures are placed behind the clamp and are not tied until the clamp is removed.

ix. The chest is closed in layers without drainage.

x. Pressures in the space are adjusted by using a Maxwell box.

89. PERICARDIECTOMY

i. Six pre-operative points:–
   - (a) Start breathing exercises before operation.
   - (b) Aspirate serous cavities and aid their clearance with diuretics.
   - (c) Start antituberculous treatment if necessary.
   - (d) Avoid excessive intravenous therapy.
   - (e) Liver damage may contraindicate drugs such as morphine.
   - (f) Start Digoxin.

ii. Median sternotomy gives adequate exposure.

iii. The internal mammary and anterior intercostal vessels are divided and ligated.

iv. A self-retaining retractor is introduced to expose the heart and its covering. The left pleural cavity is opened.

v. The phrenic nerve is dissected free.

vi. In the first instance a cruciate incision is made through the pericardium of the left ventricle, which is then freed of this covering by dissecting up the flaps but preserving the branches of the left coronary artery. The dissection stops at the atrioventricular ring.

vii. A flap can be sutured down over an accidental tear; therefore preserve the flaps, attached at their bases, until the end of the dissection.

viii. The right ventricle is freed similarly, and includes the inferior vena cava. The pleura is closed and a drain is connected to an underwater seal. The intercostal layer is repaired.

ix. The pectoral muscle is re-sutured.

x. The chest is closed.

90. PERSISTENT DUCTUS ARTERIOSUS

i. The child is placed in the lateral position, left side uppermost.

ii. The chest is opened through the fourth interspace or rib bed.

iii. The aorta is identified, and the mediastinal pleura is divided around the lateral border of the arch and the flap is reflected medially which lifts up the vagus and recurrent nerves which pass between the duct and the aorta.

iv. The duct is identified by its thrill, and the aorta above and below is encircled by loose tapes to facilitate emergency clamping.

v. The duct is dissected free then divided and sutured or doubly ligated.

vi. The lung is expanded and the chest drained employing an underwater seal.

vii. The chest wall and skin are closed.

viii. The duct in adults may be calcified or aneurysmal, its closure must be approached with caution.

91. PULMONARY/SYSTEMIC ANASTOMOSES

Palliative or first-stage procedures in severe cyanotic heart disease may be established and are designed to increase pulmonary blood flow. Total correction in infancy would render these operations obsolete.

Blalock/Taussig (Subclavian pulmonary artery)

i. The child is placed in the lateral position, right side uppermost (A left-sided Blalock may exceptionally be indicated).

ii. The chest is opened through the right fourth rib bed or intercostal space.

iii. The full length of the right main pulmonary artery is mobilised and secured proximally and distally with "snares" of suitably thick silk which are left loose.

iv. The full lengths of innominate, right subclavian and right carotid arteries are mobilised in the thorax, with division of the subclavian branches. The ansa subclavia and the right recurrent laryngeal nerve are preserved.

v. The subclavian artery is lightly clamped, divided distally and swung down to the pulmonary artery which is lightly snared.

vi. End-to-side anastomosis is performed with a continuous suture. The clamp and snares are removed as soon as possible.

vii. The chest is closed with underwater drainage.

*N.B.–The Blalock-*Hanlon *operation involves the creation of an atrial septal defect to cause blood mixing at atrial level. The two procedures should not be confused.*

Waterston (Aorto/Pulmonary Anastomosis)

i. The approach is as for a right Blalock-Taussig as in i., ii., iii., above.

ii. The azygos vein is divided, the superior vena cava partly mobilised and retracted anteriorly. The pericardium is opened behind the cava to expose the ascending aorta.

iii. A DeBakey/Cooley angled clamp is so applied as to clamp the pulmonary artery but anteriorly to include a portion of the aorta within its jaws.

iv. A 3 mm incision is made in both vessels and side-to-side anastomosis is performed with a continuous suture.

v. After removal of the clamp the chest is closed with underwater drainage.

PULMONARY ARTERY BANDING

Where, due to intracardiac shunts pulmonary blood flow is excessive, it may be reduced by banding.

This manoeuvre is usually an adjunct to others such as ligation of ductus so that the approach already exists.

i. The main pulmonary trunk between the valve and the bifurcation is encircled with a nylon tape.

ii. Under continuous E.C.G. and pressure monitoring the tape is tightened to the desired degree and secured with sutures.

92. COARCTATION OF AORTA

i. Endotracheal anaesthesia is used. A stable drip is established.

ii. The patient lies in the lateral position, left side uppermost.

iii. The chest is opened through the fifth rib bed. Large thin-walled collateral vessels, in latissimus dorsi should be ligated not coagulated.

iv. The lung is retracted to expose the left subclavian artery and the aorta.

v. The mediastinal pleura is divided and reflected from the root of the left subclavian artery to well below the coarctation, with the division of the left superior intercostal vein. Vagus and recurrent nerves are preserved.

vi. The aorta is freely mobilised over this area, carefully dividing only those intercostal arteries nearest the coarctation.

vii. Clamps are applied and the coarcted segment is excised. With a short coarctation end-to-end anastomosis is performed, with a long one a woven Dacron prosthesis is interposed. A continuous everting suture is employed.

viii. The chest is closed with an under-water seal.

93. CLOSED MITRAL VALVOTOMY

i. Controlled respiration anaesthesia is used. A stable drip is established.

ii. The patient lies in the lateral position, left side uppermost.

iii. The chest is opened through the fifth rib bed and the lung is retracted posteriorly.

iv. The heart is exposed by dividing the pericardium 1 cm in front of the phrenic nerve.

v. Purse string sutures are inserted around the base of the left atrial appendage and at the apex of the left ventricle.

vi. The atrial appendage is clamped and a finger's width incision is made in its lateral wall. The clamp is momentarily released to wash out loose clot.

vii. The index finger is inserted to explore the valve and a ventriculotomy within the apical purse-string allows introduction of a Tubbs Dilator which is guided through the valve by the finger. Progressive dilatation reduces risks of regurgitation.

viii. The carotid arteries should be temporarily compressed by the anaesthetist if passage of clots is threatened.

ix. At completion, the atrial appendage is excised and the purse-string is reinforced with a continuous suture. The ventriculotomy is closed with a cross-stitch.

x. Check and clear vessels for emboli.

xi. The pericardium is loosely closed with a few interrupted sutures.

xii. The chest is closed with underwater drainage.

94. THYMECTOMY

i. Controlled respiration is used.

ii. The chest is opened by a median sternotomy.

iii. The thymus is an 'H' shaped structure and its limbs may extend as low as the diaphragm and as high as the neck. It is progressively dissected free throughout its full extent, ligating vessels as encountered.

iv. An anterior mediastinal drain is inserted.

v. The sternum is closed with stainless steel wire.

vi. The chest is closed.

95. STRICTURE OF OESOPHAGUS

i. Diagnosis is suggested by contrast radiography and confirmed by oesophagoscopy.

ii. Dilate the stricture.

iii. The treatment depends on the following factors, the pathology, the rigidity of the stricture, the presence of a hiatus hernia, the length of the involved segment, the age and the general condition of the patient.

iv. For conservative control of a simple stricture, the patient may be instructed in swallowing mercury bougies, or may be admitted at intervals for dilatation.

v. For carcinoma excision or intubation with a Mousseau-Barbin or Celestin tube is undertaken.

vi. Hiatus hernia treatment is discussed later.

vii. The stricture may be excised and the defect bridged using stomach, jejunum or colon, Pyloroplasty and Pyloromyotomy is then added.

96. CARCINOMA OF THE OESOPHAGUS

Left-sided Thoraco-abdominal approach for lower half of Oesophagus

i. Controlled respiration anaesthesia, intravenous drip, and diathermy are used.

ii. A thoraco-abdominal approach is made through the eighth rib bed.

iii. The diaphragm is divided down to the oesophageal hiatus.

iv. The left pulmonary ligament is divided.

v. The mediastinal pleura is divided and the oesophagus and growth mobilised.

vi. The stomach is freed by dividing the gastrocolic omentum and the vasa brevia; the right gastric and the right gastroepiploic vessels are preserved.

vii. A pyloromyotomy is performed (Rammstedt).

viii. The stomach is divided below the cardia and along the lesser curve to fashion a tube.

ix. The oesophagus is divided above the growth and removed.

x. The proximal end of the oesophagus is anastomosed to the fundus of the stomach. Linen or steel wire may be used. The strong layer of the oesophagus is the mucosa.*

xi. The stomach is anchored to the pleura.*

xii. The anastomosis may be covered by a flap of pleura.

xiii. The lung is re-expanded.

xiv. A water-seal drain is inserted and the diaphragm and wound closed.

The upper half of the thoracic oesophagus is approached through the right sixth rib bed following laparotomy and mobilisation of stomach. The anastomosis is done on the right side of the chest.

97. POSTERIOR APPROACH FOR SUBPHRENIC ABSCESS

i. General or local anaesthesia is employed.

ii. The patient lies on his sound side, or sits up with his arms supported. A chest X-ray exhibited in theatre confirms the presence of a twelfth rib.

iii. The incision is made along the line of the twelfth rib and deepened to include its periosteum.

iv. The rib is removed subperiostally.

v. The subcostal vessels and nerve are ligated and divided.

vi. A horizontal incision is now made across the rib bed to avoid opening the pleura.

vii. The abscess is found by blunt dissection, and drained.

98. DIAPHRAGMATIC HERNIA

Two Approaches

Through the Chest. (Sliding Hiatus Hernia).

i. A Ryle's tube is present in the stomach.

ii. The patient is placed in the lateral position with the head-end of the table lowered.

iii. The left chest is opened through the eighth rib or interspace, the pulmonary ligament is divided and the lung retracted to expose the region of the oesophageal hiatus.

iv. The oesophagus is freely mobilised from the hiatus to the inferior pulmonary vein.

v. The crura are carefully defined and the hiatus is freed.

vi. Three or four double-ended sutures are placed at the oesophagogastric junction and the ends are then passed carefully through the hiatus to pierce the diaphragm from below upwards at the margins of the crura. Traction on these sutures reduces the hernia and they are then tied.

vii. The crura are tightened behind the oesophagus by three or four interrupted sutures leaving just sufficient room for the tip of the index finger to pass alongside the oesophagus.

viii. The chest is drained to an underwater seal.

Through the chest. (Para-oesophageal Hernia).

i. The approach and mobilisation are as for sliding hernia.

ii. The stomach prolapses into the chest alongside the oesophagus and carries with it a large sac. The sac is excised and the stomach reduced into the abdomen.

iii. The hiatus is reconstituted by approximating the crura with as many interrupted sutures as necessary.

iv. The chest is closed with underwater drainage.

Through the Abdomen

i. General anaesthesia is used; a Ryle's tube is present in the oesophagus.

ii. The abdomen is opened through a high left paramedian incision.

iii. The great advantage of this approach is that a careful laparotomy may be performed. A peptic ulcer of the stomach or duodenum – with or without early pyloric stenosis – gall stones, or even a carcinoma may be discovered, all requiring priority in the patient's treatment. However peptic strictures cannot be dealt with through this approach.

iv. The hiatus is exposed and the left lobe of the liver mobilised by dividing the triangular ligament.

v. The oesophagus, stomach and sac are mobilised.

vi. The sac is excised.

vii. The crura are brought together in front or behind the oesophagus to reduce the hiatus to a size allowing the admission of the tip of an index finger. Non-absorbable material is used, and the suture includes the phrenooesophageal ligament cuff left on the oesophagus.*

viii. The peritoneum is repaired.

ix. The wound is closed.

99. RADICAL MASTECTOMY (Halsted)

i. General anaesthesia. Diathermy is used, therefore avoid an inflammable anaesthetic.

ii. The arm is held at right angles to the body on an arm board or suspended from a drip stand by a sling about the wrist. Care is taken to avoid traction injuries of the brachial plexus.

iii. Define the margins of the growth. Make an elliptical incision including the nipple, the skin over the growth, and 5 cm of normal skin beyond its margin.* Extend the incision upwards up to the shoulder to cover the insertion of the pectoralis major tendon. Extend the inision medially and downwards towards a point on the opposite* side of the midline midway between the ensiform cartilage and the umbilicus. Avoid placing the upper part of the incision along the inferior margin of the anterior axillary fold, as a "bridle-scar" develops.

iv. Deepen the skin incision and reflect the lateral and medial flaps including a small amount of subcutaneous fat. Approximately half the subcutaneous fat is left on the skin, and the thinner the patient, the greater care is required to avoid cutting into the breast tissue, which is recognised by its white colour. Mobilise the lateral flap as far back as the anterior border of Latissimus dorsi. Mobilise the upper half of the medial flap to beyond the medial end of the clavicle.

v. Identify the cephalic vein by sharp dissection so that it can be preserved.

vi. Cut* a hole in the axillary fascia to permit passage of a finger below the insertion of the pectoralis tendon, and bring out the finger below the cephalic vein so that it embraces the tendon.

vii. Divide the tendon close to the bone to avoid the remnants adhering to the scar.

viii. Further mobilise the pectoralis major by sharp dissection along its upper border, dividing it at its clavicular origin and continuing this mobilisation to expose the medial aspects of the first two intercostal spaces. Branches of the acromiothoracic vessels are found and with the pectoral nerves, are divided. This procedure reveals the pectoralis minor and its fascia.

ix. Divide the pectoralis minor tendon immediately below its coracoid insertion and the fascia on either side. The axillary vessels and nerves together with their covering fascial sheath are exposed.

x. The axilla is then dissected from the side of the axillary vein proceeding medially, and from the apex of the axilla passing downwards by a combination of sharp and blunt dissection. The knife, the dissecting scissors, finger covered by gauze, Lahey swabs and blunt dissecting forceps all have their uses. The small vein tributaries of the axillary vein are cleared and divided a quarter of an inch* from the main vein. These veins are ligated carefully to avoid air embolus.

xi. The nerves to Latissimus dorsi and serratus anterior are preserved, and note that the nerve to Latissimus is found near the subscapular vessels and on a more superficial plane than the other nerve. The nerves may be sacrificed if involved glands are found to be adherent to them.

xii. The breast is excised from the chest wall, clipping the lateral and anterior perforating branches before division. The excision of the mass of tissue is carried to the opposite side of the midline, and includes the upper part of the rectus sheath.

xiii. The rest of the medial flap still attached is now mobilised to complete the excision.

xiv. Careful haemostasis is obtained and an immediate skin graft is applied, if necessary, to avoid suturing under tension.

xv. A suction tube is left in for four days.

Conservative radical mastectomy (Patey)

The dissection may be performed preserving pectoralis major and its nerve supply but excising pectoralis minor to facilitate the axillary gland clearance.

CHAPTER X

SYMPATHECTOMY

100. Lumbar Sympathectomy
101. Upper Thoracic Sympathectomy (Anterior Approach)
102. Upper Thoracic Sympathectomy (Posterior Approach)

100. LUMBAR SYMPATHECTOMY

i. General anaesthesia is used.

ii. The flank is exposed by tilting the patient towards the opposite side, placing a sandbag behind the shoulder and buttock.

iii. An oblique or transverse incision is made.

iv. The muscles are split or divided to expose the extraperitoneal fat.

v. The peritoneal sac is raised by blunt dissection from the lateral and posterior abdominal walls to uncover the medial margin of the psoas muscle and the aorta or inferior vena, depending on the side.

vi. Five structures – ureters,* obturator nerve, gonadal vessels, inferior mesenteric vein and duodenum – may be seen. Retractors are inserted.

vii. The obturator nerve has no ganglia, and is easily identified.

viii. The sympathetic chain and ganglia, lying medial to the psoas muscle, are more easily felt than seen. The chain is exposed by dissecting through the overlying fascia.

ix. The chain is picked up with forceps and dissected upwards and downwards, exposing the second and third lumbar ganglia. The first right lumbar ganglion lies deep to the duodenum. The fourth lies behind the common iliac vessels.

x. Divide the chain, removing approximately 5–7 cm containing two to four ganglia. Removal of Lumbar I bilaterally makes the sympathectomy more certain, but may result in loss of ejaculation.

xi. Lumbar veins may cross the chain and are clipped with Cushing's silver clips. Pack the area for five minutes if accidental tearing occurs.

xii. The muscles are sutured.

xiii. The skin is closed.

101. UPPER THORACIC SYMPATHECTOMY
Anterior Approach

i. Controlled respiration anaesthesia is employed.

ii. A sandbag is placed between the shoulders, and the head is turned to the opposite side.

iii. A skin crease incision is made one finger-breadth above the medial half of the clavicle.

iv. The incision is deepened through the platysma to expose the deep fascia.

v. Dissect out and divide the external jugular vein, then divide the clavicular head of the sternomastoid. The muscle may consist of two layers.

vi. The next landmark is the omohyoid muscle and its fascia; this muscle is divided.

vii. Next identify the transverse cervical vessels and trace the artery medially. It will lead to the phrenic nerve, which it crosses.

viii. Mobilise the phrenic nerve from beneath the prevertebral fascia and draw it aside on a tape.

ix. The scalenus anterior can be felt with the finger as a tight band.

x. If in the way, the thyrocervical trunk may be mobilised and divided. Note that collateral vessels may require saving.

xi. Mobilise the scalenus anterior down to the first rib, and divide it at its insertion, preserving the medial part of it on the left side to avoid damaging the thoracic duct.

xii. In the next layer is the subclavian artery, and this mobilises very easily by blunt dissection. A rubber catheter is introduced round it to act as a sling.

xiii. Identify the inner border of the first rib, and detach Sibson's fascia from it with the finger. Alternatively, Lahey swabs may be used.

xiv. Expose the necks of the first three ribs by Lahey swab dissection.

xv. Identify the sympathetic chain with the index finger* and clear off the overlying fascia. A lighted retractor is inserted, together with two other small reflecting retractors, and the chain is seen.

xvi. At the neck of the first rib there are three structures present from medial to lateral – the sympathetic nerve, the superior intercostal vessels, and the first thoracic nerve.

xvii. The chain is divided below the third ganglion, and dissected up by dividing its communication as far as the first thoracic ganglion, which is left to avoid Horner's Syndrome.

xviii The end is buried in the scalenus anterior.

xix. The sternomastoid and platysma are repaired and the skin approximated with clips.

xx. An angled silver clip applicator is of great help in dealing with small vessels that cross the nerve or its ganglia.

102. UPPER THORACIC SYMPATHECTOMY
Posterior Approach

i. Controlled respiration anaesthesia is used. Pneumothorax may occur accidentally during or after the operation. An adequate light is required – head light or lighted retractor.

ii. The prone position is used. A pillow is placed under the chest.

iii. A vertical 7 cm incision is made centred over the third rib, 5 cm from midline opposite the second spine.

iv. Deepen the incision down to the periosteum.

v. The periosteum is divided, stripped back and a portion of the rib removed. To aid the exposure, remove the transverse process.

vi. The pleura is seen. It is easily torn at this stage.

vii. Dissect out the intercostal nerve running under the third rib, divide it at the lateral aspect of the wound and follow it medially to find the sympathetic chain which lies anteriorly.

viii. If the exposure is difficult, remove the second rib in a similar fashion.

ix. After identifying the sympathetic chain medially, draw out the anterior and posterior roots of the intercostal nerve and divide them, cutting the posterior root medial to the posterior root ganglion. Repeat with second nerve. Notice that this may be dangerous in a post-fixed brachial plexus.

x. Divide the sympathetic chain below its third ganglion, dissect up the chain to the first ganglion by dividing all the branches and cover the end with silk, then bury it.

xi. Allow the muscles to fall back, draw together and sew up skin.

CHAPTER XI

UROLOGY

103. Cystoscopy and Ureteric Catheterisation
104. Nephrectomy
105. Partial Nephrectomy
106. Pyelolithotomy
107. Nephrolithotomy
108. Nephro-ureterectomy
109. Nephrectomy Right Abdominal Nephrectomy and Adrenalectomy
110. Left Abdominal Nephrectomy and Adrenalectomy
111. Hydronephrosis
112. Exposures of Ureter
113. Removing Ureteric Stone through Bladder
114. Transplantation of Ureters
115. Coffey I Method
116. Cordonnier's Method
117. The Ileal Bladder
118. Diagnosis of Carcinoma of Bladder
119. Treatment of Carcinoma of Bladder
120. Partial Cystectomy
121. Total Cystectomy and Transplantation of Ureters
122. Suprapubic Cystostomy
123. Transvescial Prostatectomy
124. Retropubic Prostatectomy
125. Partial Amputation of Penis
126. Total Amputation of Penis and Bilateral Orchidectomy
127. Hypospadias
128. Diverticulectomy (Bladder)
129. Litholapaxy
130. Hydrocele Operations
131. Strictures of Urethra
132. Ruptured Urethra
133. Orchidectomy
134. Epididymectomy

135 Abdominal Hysterectomy

103. CYSTOSCOPY AND URETERIC CATHETERISATION

i. The patient empties his bladder and lies supine, or is set up in the lithotomy position. General or local anaesthesia is used.

ii. If supine, a sandbag is placed under the sacrum and the legs are abducted and the heels supported on a board placed across the end of the table.

iii. Metal sounds are available and are employed if difficulty is encountered passing the instrument.

iv. Check the transformer and ensure the dial is at zero.

v. Look through the telescope and clean lens if necessary.

vi. Uretric catheters and their stylettes are checked and lubricated.

vii. Insert the telescope and make sure catheters will pass.

viii. Switch on the current and adjust light. It changes from yellow to white.

ix. Check that the water is at 38°C in the reservoir, connect up and wash out the air bubbles. Sterilise the urethral orifice with swab soaked in antiseptic.

x. Lubricate and pass the cystoscope, remove the telescope, empty and measure residual urine. Send a specimen for pathological examination if required.

xi. Wash out bladder until water is crystal clear.

xii. Leave in 200 ml of water.

xiii. Examine the bladder, its ureteric orifices, and its neck. The presence of infection, stones, tumours, diverticula, prostatic enlargement, trabeculation etc. are noted.

xiv. With the aid of the ureteric guide (Albarran-lever), pass the catheters and remove the stylettes.

xv. Ensure the ureteric guide is in the "down" position, empty the bladder and with the telescope in position remove the cystoscope leaving the ureteric catheters *in situ*.

xvi. The catheter ends are put into sterile test-tubes that are strapped to the thigh.

xvii. A urinary antibiotic may be given for the following five days as minor traumata always occur.

104. NEPHRECTOMY
Posterior Approach

i. Check the function of the other kidney.

ii. General anaesthesia is employed. The bladder is emptied. Abdominal X-ray is in Theatre.

iii. The patient lies on the sound side, and the leg on that side* is well flexed. The opposite arm is held forward by placing it on a Carter-Braine rest. The table may be split to widen the area between the ribs and iliac crest, or a loin rest may be used. A wide strap around the patient's pelvis and the table helps stability.

iv. An oblique incision is made, commencing over the neck of the twelfth rib – check the site of this rib by X-ray. The incision runs forward between the rib margin and the iliac crest and may be extended up to or beyond the lateral margin of the rectus sheath.

v. The access is improved posteriorly by removing the twelfth rib subperiosteally. The following structures are preserved; pleura, subcostal nerve, colon and peritoneum.

vi. The incision is deepened to expose the latissimus dorsi and the external oblique, and these muscles are divided and split respectively.

vii. The internal oblique and transversus muscles and transversalis fascia are divided to expose the extraperitoneal fat.

viii. Posteriorly, by dividing vertically all laminae of the lumbar fascia, the twelfth rib, if not already removed, may be mobilised.

ix. The peritoneum is mobilised forwards by blunt dissection to expose the fascia of Zuckerkandl.

x. The fascia is opened and the kidney seen.

xi. If possible, it is brought out of the wound; if not, a self-retaining retractor is inserted to aid further dissection.

xii. The ureter is identified and transected. (In certain cases it is excised completely.)

xiii. The renal vessels are triply clamped and divided between the middle and distal clamp.

xiv. The wound is drained.

xv. The muscles are sutured together with interrupted sutures that are tied after removing the kidney rest, or straightening the table.

105. PARTIAL NEPHRECTOMY

i. The kidney is exposed and delivered. It is secured by a tape encircling the pedicle.

ii. The vessels at the hilum are gently dissected, and if a distinct blood supply is found for the part to be removed, it is ligated and divided.

iii. The hilar vessels are controlled by the assistant's fingers.

iv. The segment is removed with its calyces and associated part of renal pelvis, leaving fringe of healthy capsule to cover the raw area.

v. Vessels are isolated and ligated, or under-run. The pelvis is repaired with plain catgut.

vi. The edges of the kidney are approximated with catgut over a graft of fat or crushed muscle.

vii. The kidney is replaced.

viii. The wound is drained.

106. PYELOLITHOTOMY

i. The renal pelvis is cleared of fat and any small vessels are under-run.

ii. It is opened posteriorly, if possible, between stay-sutures longitudinally or transversely; the stone is removed with stone-forceps. The small wound is then closed with catgut.

iii. If infected, the renal pelvis may be drained with a tube (pyelostomy).

107. NEPHROLITHOTOMY

i. A stone inaccessible through the pelvis may be localised by inserting two needles at right angles to one another at the possible site and then X-raying the kidney. Repeat until the stone is localised.

ii. It is approached through Brodel's line which lies 1·0 cm behind the convex margin of the kidney (or a radial incision). The hilar vessels are controlled during this procedure again by the assistant's fingers.

iii. The stone is removed, haemostasis is secured and a check X-ray is performed. Selected renal cooling allows prolongation of operative time with a bloodless field.

iv. If uninfected the wound is closed; if not, a drainage tube may be left down through the kidney into the renal pelvis (nephrostomy).

v. A wide exposure of the posterior aspect of the pelvis is achieved by dissecting medially over its surface and retracting the kidney substance (Gilles-Vernet).

108. NEPHRO-URETERECTOMY

i. This operation may be extremely difficult if the inflammation and subsequent fibrosis has spread outside the kidney. The most difficult part is the mobilisation of the kidney, so this should be performed first.

ii. The following structures may require to be separated from the right kidney – liver, diaphragm and suprarenal, duodenum and colon; and on the left side – stomach, spleen and colon.

iii. The ureter if readily found may be followed to identify the kidney hilum.

iv. After mobilisation of the kidney and division of its vessels, the ureter is mobilised as far down as possible, and the kidney pushed down behind the peritoneum, or the kidney may be left outside the wound anchored by the ureter, and the wound sutured and drained.

v. The lower end of the ureter is approached through a vertical incision in the lower abdomen. The peritoneum is stripped back, the inferior vesical vessels are carefully divided, and the ureter is removed, allowing a sufficient length attached to the bladder to hold a ligature. The kidney is removed with the ureter, or if the kidney has been left outside the upper wound the ureter is drawn through the upper wound from above, after carbolising and covering the end of the ureter. The ureter may be divided flush with the bladder and its intramural part diathermized if complete mucosal destruction is required. A drain is then left at the site of the division of the ureter and brought out of the lower wound.

109. NEPHRECTOMY

Five indications for abdominal nephrectomy

i. A very large tumour.

ii. A tumour of doubtful operability. The liver may be found full of secondaries or other structures may be found extensively involved.

iii. Following multiple abdominal injuries.

iv. For hypernephromata so that the renal vein may be clamped and divided before disturbing the kidney.

v. Possibly to check on the presence of the other kidney, if not checked previously. Its presence does not signify function.

109a. RIGHT ABDOMINAL NEPHRECTOMY

i. General anaesthesia is used.

ii. The abdomen is opened through a right paramedian incision, and explored.

iii. The hepatic flexure is mobilised by dividing its attachments, and packed off downwards and medially along with the small intestine.

iv. The second part of the duodenum is held over to the left and the peritoneum along its right border divided. By this procedure the duodenum and head of the pancreas can be mobilised as far as the inferior vena cava (Kocher's manoeuvre).

v. The fascia of the kidney is then exposed, picked up and divided. The hilar vessels and ureter are divided and ligated and the kidney is mobilised and removed.

109b. RIGHT ABDOMINAL ADRENALECTOMY

i.-iv. Similar steps are carried out as in right abdominal nephrectomy.

v. Traction on the kidney brings down the adrenal gland.

vi. Its exposure is facilitated by extending the incision in the posterior parietal peritoneum upwards and retracting the right lobe of the liver (Barlow).

vii. The adrenal veins are clipped with Cushing silver clips and divided.

viii. Blunt dissection mobilises the gland for its removal.

ix. Accessory glands may require removal.

110. LEFT ABDOMINAL NEPHRECTOMY AND APPROACH TO THE LEFT ADRENAL GLAND

i. General anaesthesia is used.

ii. The abdomen is opened by a long left paramedian incision, and explored.

iii. The incision may be extended transversely if the patient is deep and broad.

iv. The spleen is held over to the left and the left leaf of the lienorenal ligament divided.

v. The hand can then be inserted behind the spleen and tail of the pancreas, and these structures can then be mobilised forwards off the posterior abdominal wall.

vi. The kidney fascia (Zuckerlandl) is then exposed, picked up and opened.

vii. The kidney is now mobilised manually, and the vessels of the hilum, and the ureter together with any extra polar vessels, can be seen and dealt with. If this approach is used for the adrenal gland, this structure is seen on the upper pole of the kidney, and is mobilised gently with blunt dissection. The large adrenal vein emptying into the left renal vein is clipped with Cushing silver clips and divided. Other vessels are similarly treated and the gland removed.

viii. The spleen is examined to ensure that no damage has occurred to it and is then replaced in the abdomen.

111. HYDRONEPHROSIS

i. The function of the opposite kidney is checked. Instrumentation before operation is avoided to prevent infection. The urine should be sterile.

ii. The kidney is explored and various procedures can be tried apart from nephrectomy, depending on the cause. One or more of the following may meet the requirements of a given case.

(a) Small arteries obstructing the ureter may be divided provided infarction is not caused. The ureter may be re-implanted to avoid such an obstruction.

(b) Adhesions between ureter and pelvis causing kinking are divided.

(c) The connective tissue surrounding the renal artery and pelvis and containing the renal nerves may be removed. Alternatively the splanchnic nerves and the first two lumbar ganglia may be excised.

(d) The kidney may be folded on itself to approximate its poles and polar vessels. (Hamilton Stewart.) This prevents contact between displaced or aberrant renal vessels and the kidney pelvis.

(e) The size of the lumen of the pelvi-ureteric junction may be increased by incising it longitudinally and sewing it up transversely; a V-Y (Foley) advancement may be effective.

(f) The pelvi-ureteric junction may be excised and the ureter re-implanted to drain the most dependent part of the renal pelvis.

(g) Redundant pelvis is excised (with other plastic procedures) to avoid stagnation.

(h) Side-to-side anastomoses between the pelvis and ureter may be established.

(i) As an alternative procedure.
The pelvi-ureteric junction and the redundant portion of the pelvis is excised leaving the lower portion of the pelvis into

which the cut ureter is anastomosed. The upper part of the divided pelvis is closed. To facilitate the implantation the upper end of the ureter is slit up for 3 cm and a ureteric catheter is left in during the procedure to ensure patency (Anderson-Hynes).
A small tube may be left down and through the ureter for two weeks or more.

(j) As a last resort a non-functioning kidney may be removed.

112. EXPOSURES OF URETER

Five points to identify Ureter

i. Characteristic vermicular movements may be seen.
ii. It crosses the commencement of the external iliac artery.
iii. It crosses the tip of the ischial spine.
iv. It is adherent to the peritoneum.
v. It is crossed by many structures, including vas and uterine artery.

Upper third

Approach as for the kidney via the lumbar route, previously described.

Lower two-thirds

i. X-ray before operating to verify position of stone. Empty the bladder.
ii. Approach extraperitoneally by a lower vertical midline or paramedian incision. Place tape above the stone to prevent losing it.
iii. If possible, the stone is disimpacted and removed through a linear incision higher up.
iv. Pass a bougie down the ureter to ensure its patency.
v. Close the ureteric opening with interrupted plain catgut sutures, and drain the wound.

Techniques for Dealing with a Divided Ureter

i. Re-anastomose the cut ends or anastomose end of divided ureter to the side of the opposite ureter.

ii. Re-implant ureter obliquely into bladder. Divide ureteric end to fashion two flaps and suture them down to the bladder mucosa.

iii. Fashion tube from bladder (Boari). A 3 cm wide flap is used. The ureter may be introduced under the vesical mucosa to produce valve-like action.

iv. Anastomose the ureter to the bowel.

v. Cutaneous ureterostomy.

113. FIVE WAYS OF REMOVING A URETERIC STONE THROUGH THE BLADDER

i. The stone may be passed following any instrumentation of the ureteric orifice, with or without injection into the ureter of lubricants or antispasmodics.

ii. By use of a loop catheter;

iii. or cork-screw (Ainsworth-Davis);

iv. or fixed metal stone basket (Johnson);

v. or by a basket that can be opened and closed (Councill).

114. TRANSPLANTATION OF URETERS

Five general principles

i. Avoid stripping with damage to the blood supply.

ii. Avoid kinking, twisting or tension.

iii. Avoid tight suturing.

iv. Haemostasis must be complete to avoid a haematoma which may compress the ureter or predispose to ascending sepsis.

v. Use the pelvic colon or rectosigmoid for implantation.

Rectosigmoid bladder

This segment may be used only for the storage of urine. Check if rectal incontinence is present. It is isolated by dividing the pelvic colon above the ureteric transplant sites, bringing out the proximal cut end as a colostomy, closing the distal end and returning it to the abdomen.

115. TRANSPLANTATION OF URETER

Coffey I Method

i. General anaesthesia; Trendelenburg position; the bladder is emptied; the bowel has been prepared.

ii. A midline or paramedian incision is made.

iii. The abdomen is opened and explored.

iv. The sigmoid colon is exposed by packing off the bowel, and a self-retaining retractor inserted.

v. The right ureter is identified and the overlying peritoneum divided.

vi. The ureter is traced downwards, minimally mobilised, ligated distally and divided obliquely.

vii. The proximal cut end is held by a catgut suture with an atraumatic needle at each end.

viii. The ureter is now held across the colon without angulation or tension to determine its lie, and this area demarcated with stay sutures.

ix. A submucous tunnel is now made by dividing the seromuscular layer.

x. A stab opening in the mucosa is made at the lower end of the trough and the ureteric anchoring sutures passed through the bowel from within outwards and tied 2·5 cm below the stab opening.

xi. The ureter is now covered by suturing together the seromuscular edges.

xii. The anchoring suture is buried.

xiii. The peritoneum is mobilised and brought over the anastomosis.

xiv. The left ureter is transplanted at a higher level.

116. TRANSPLANTATION OF URETER

Cordonnier's Method

i. Cordonnier emphasises bringing the bowel to the ureter.*

ii. The ureter is divided and the proximal end anchored to the bowel by a silk stay-suture placed 1 cm above the cut end.

iii. The bowel is opened longitudinally and the ureter anastomosed to the bowel, mucosa to mucosa with catgut. The sutures pass through the whole thickness of the ureter.

iv. The adventia of the ureter is sutured to the serosa of the bowel.

v. The area of the anastomosis is fixed to the parietes, covered with the peritoneum and the sigmoid rolled downwards to produce straightening of the ureter.

117. THE ILEAL BLADDER

i. General anaesthesia is employed, the bowel is prepared. Trendelenburg position may be useful.

ii. The abdomen is opened through a lower left paramedian incision and explored.

iii. The bowel is packed off to expose the lower ileum and pelvis. A self-retaining retractor is helpful.

iv. A loop of ileum 30 cm long with its distal end not nearer than 25 cm from the caecum* is chosen.

v. The ureters are identified and the position for anastomosis to the proximal end of the ileal loop decided upon. The left may be placed 2·5 cm from the end and the right 5 cm beyond. There must be no tension on the suture lines.

vi. The bowel loop is prepared by dividing the mesentery so as to preserve an adequate blood supply, and allowing the loop to be placed in its final position without tension.

vii. The bowel is divided between soft clamps. A Cope's crushing clamp is used on the distal end of the isolated loop to facilitate its passage through the anterior abdominal wall.

viii. The continuity of the ileum is restored by performing an end-to-end anastomosis in front of the isolated loop.

ix. The opening in the mesentery is closed.

x. The proximal end of the loop is closed.

xi. The ureters are exposed below. The distal ends are ligated. The proximal ends are mobilised to provide adequate length and brought out through small openings in the peritoneum above and implanted or anastomosed to the ileum along the antimesenteric border at the predetermined points.

xii. The pelvic peritoneum is repaired.

xiii. The ileum is brought out through a stab wound in the right iliac fossa. It may lie extraperitoneally or transperitoneally, in which case the lateral space must be closed.

xiv. The mucosa is sutured to the edge of the skin of the stab wound.

118. CYSTOSCOPIC AIDS TO DIAGNOSIS OF CARCINOMA OF THE BLADDER

Ten points

i. The urine and the bladder wall are infected.*

ii. The tumour may have ulcerated.

iii. There may be phosphatic debris on the surface of the tumour.

iv. The fronds may appear thicker than the delicate branches of a simple papilloma.

v. The fronds may have fused.

vi. The bladder wall adjacent to the growth may show small deposits, some oedema, bullae or puckering.

vii. The tumour bleeds readily when touched.

viii. It may be pushed with an electrode to demonstrate the attachment of the tumour to the bladder wall. The electrode may be made to adhere to the growth by commencing diathermy destruction, and then by pulling on the electrode a better view of the base of the growth and its mobility may be obtained.

ix. Anything that does not appear as a delicate frond-like structure should be considered as malignant, and a biopsy taken.

x. Care should be exercised, however, in distinguishing a stone covered by necrotic material.

119. TREATMENT OF CARCINOMA OF THE BLADDER

There are a variety of treatments, and below is a list:

i. Transurethral coagulation: An attempt is made to destroy the entire tumour on the first occasion.

ii. Transvesical coagulation: Protect the wound edges by using towels soaked in 1:1000 silver nitrate and destroy the tumour under vision.

iii. Partial cystectomy: It is difficult to judge the extent of spread; dissemination of growth may follow the operation. The tumour may have a multifocal origin, and involvement of both ureters or the internal meatus of the bladder contraindicates this treatment.

iv. Total cystectomy with transplantation of ureters: The cystectomy may be performed as a radical or palliative procedure.

v. Transplantation of ureters as a palliative procedure.

vi. Introduction of Radon seeds transvesically, or introduction of Radon seeds into the growth from within and without.

vii. Irradiation through the open bladder.

viii. Introduction of radium needles, or wire.

ix. Deep X-ray therapy, with or without the transplantation of ureters.

x. Introduction of radio-active fluids or cytotoxic drugs.

120. PARTIAL CYSTECTOMY

General remarks

The operation is rarely performed owing to a high local recurrence rate. However, a painful lesion is removed, and the results of more radical treatments of the malignant bladder are not yet encouraging.

Technique

i. The bladder is washed out with silver nitrate.

ii. Position: The patient is fixed for Trendelenburg tilt, and tilted if exposure is thereby improved.

iii. An incision is made in the midline, or transversely.

iv. The peritoneum is opened and a laparotomy performed. The bladder is then opened extraperitoneally and with diathermy the growth and a 2·5 cm margin of healthy tissue, and any adherent peritoneum, are excised.
The bladder is reconstituted and any openings in the peritoneum are closed. A catheter is left in the bladder, and a drainage tube at the site of bladder repair.

v. If the ureter requires division, it is subsequently re-implanted into the bladder by employing the following technique: The end is split at opposite poles for 0·5 cm, the ureter taken through a new opening in the bladder, and the two portions opened and sutured to the bladder mucosa.

121. TOTAL CYSTECTOMY AND TRANSPLANTATION OF URETERS

i. The patient is placed for Trendelenburg tilt; diathermy is ready and an intravenous drip in position.

ii. The abdomen is opened through a long right paramedian incision extending down to the pubis.

iii. The peritoneum is opened and explored for secondaries, glands and peritoneal involvement. Any area of adherent or involved peritoneum is removed with the bladder. The uterus and part of the vaginal wall may be excised if implication is present or suspected. Glands along the internal iliac vessels are removed with the bladder.

iv. A self-retaining retractor is inserted, the small bowel packed off and the table is tilted. The anterior division of the internal iliac artery is tied on both sides.

v. The ureters are now identified and divided low down.

vi. The upper end is held with a stay suture, the lower end with a cholecystectomy forceps.

vii. The extraperitoneal dissection commences by identifying the "key" structure – the vas deferens (Grey Turner). It is divided and traced down along the lateral aspect of the bladder. Five structures are dealt with as one proceeds – the obliterated hypogastric vessels, superior and inferior vesical vessels, lateral vesical ligaments and the arteries to the seminal vesicles.

viii. The urachus is divided and held. The dissection of the bladder continues to expose the apex of the prostate.

ix. The seminal vesicles are now identified, and in order to enter the Space of Denonvilliers, the fascia behind them is divided with scissors.

x. The space is developed by blunt dissection and the rectum is thereby freed.

xi. The puboprostatic ligaments are divided and the urethra clamped and cut across.

xii. The bladder, vesicles, prostate, ureter stumps and iliac glands are then removed.

xiii. The ureters are transplanted.

xiv. The peritoneum is reconstituted.

xv. The wound is closed with drainage.

122. SUPRA-PUBIC CYSTOSTOMY

i. General or local anaesthesia is used.

ii. General principle is to place drainage tube as high as possible* and to carry out the minimum mobilisation of the bladder to facilitate a possible prostatectomy later when the patient is fitter. A site may be selected midway between umbilicus and symphysis pubis or above.

iii. If a catheter can be passed, wash out the bladder until return is clear, and leave in 250 ml or more.

iv. A small vertical or transverse incision is made and deepened through the midline.

v. The bladder is identified by the veins and muscle on its surface.

vi. Strip up the peritoneum and extraperitoneal fat.

vii. Insert two stay-sutures, open the bladder, suck out the fluid. The bladder is explored.*

viii. Introduce a self-retaining catheter and close the bladder with plain catgut around the tube.

ix. Close the rectus and skin with interrupted sutures.

x. Anchor the tube to the skin so that it is not pulled out.

xi. If the tube is inserted so deeply as to impinge on the trigone, pain will be experienced at the tip of the penis.

xii. Test the flow of the tube to ensure its patency.

Note – Occasionally the operation is a "blind" one – a tube being inserted through a stab wound employing a catheter and introducer (Riches).

123. TRANSVESICAL PROSTATECTOMY

i. A catheter is passed and the bladder filled with sterile water (250 ml).

ii. A transverse (or vertical midline) abdominal incision is made. The rectus sheath is divided transversely (or vertically) and the sheath reflected upwards and downward to expose the recti, which are divided and separated to expose the extraperitoneal fat and the filmy transversalis fascia over the bladder.

iii. The fascia transversalis is divided transversely and the peritoneum and extraperitoneal fat stripped upwards to expose the bladder. The veins on the surface of the bladder help in its identification.

iv. Open the bladder between stay sutures and explore it for tumours, stones, or diverticula. If a true diverticulum is to be dealt with it is excised before enucleating the prostatic adenoma.*

v. The end of the catheter is transfixed with a long thread and held up out of the bladder.

vi. A self-retaining bladder retractor is inserted and a V-shaped area of the trigone marked out for removal with diathermy after identification of ureteric orifices. The apex of the "V" lies in the Mercier's bar between the ureteric orifices.

vii. The retractor is removed and the prostate enucleated with the index finger. If difficulty is encountered or if the patient is fat and deep, a finger of the other hand in the rectum can be most helpful.

viii. Three spheres of tissue are removed, the two lateral and the middle lobes. The method employed is to insert the finger through the internal meatus, split the commissure and gain the correct plane by compressing the gland against the pubis, then by pressure split the planes around the other lobes. The urethra is divided on the under surface of the spheres with the finger (or under vision with scissors).

ix. The bladder retractor is now inserted and a wedge of the trigone removed,* or a cut is made at three and nine o'clock (internal sphincterotomy). A volsellum forceps is useful to hold the lip of the trigone.

x. Haemostasis is obtained, aided by the insertion of posterolateral sutures. Harris' Boomerang needle is well adapted to inserting these haemostatic sutures.

xi. The catheter held by a stay-suture is drawn back into the bladder. The ends of the stay-suture holding the catheter are brought out through the bladder and abdominal wall and fixed with gauze or Emesay button at two points. The bladder is closed with three layers of plain catgut. An outer layer which does not penetrate the bladder mucosa may be of chromic gut. If bleeding is uncontrollable, the cavity may be packed with surgical haemostatic substances, or the cavity may be packed for forty-eight hours with 5 cm gauze which is brought out through a suprapubic tube. 100 ml of potassium citrate solution is left in the bladder.

xii. The space of Retzius is drained, the rectus repaired and the skin closed.

xiii. The vasa sometimes are divided and ligated at the neck of the scrotum.

xiv. A check is made to ensure that the catheter is flowing satisfactorily, and continuous drainage is established.

124. RETROPUBIC PROSTATECTOMY

i. Cystoscopy is performed first.

ii. The bladder is emptied.

iii. The transverse incision and approach is employed.

iv. The fascia transversalis is divided and the bladder separated from the pubis to expose the prostatic capsule. A self-retaining retractor is inserted.

v. Two lateral packs may be inserted one on each side to aid exposure.

vi. The veins running over the prostate are ligated.

vii. A transverse (or vertical) cut is now made through the capsule and into the "white" of the adenoma.

viii. The cut capsule edges are held and the adenoma dissected out with scissors curved on the flat. The urethra is divided under vision. The adenomatous tissue is removed, level with the surface of the adenoma.

ix. A generous wedge is now removed from the posterior lip of the bladder. Two fingers may be inserted through the bladder-neck.

x. Tags are removed and posterolateral sutures introduced and haemostasis achieved.

xi. A catheter, whistle-tipped, or a three-way Foley catheter is passed into the bladder and citrate (120 ml) introduced.

xii. The prostatic capsule is closed with plain catgut.

xiii. The packs are removed and the rectus and skin closed with a small drain in the space of Retzius.

125. PARTIAL AMPUTATION OF THE PENIS

i. General anaesthesia is used.

ii. A rubber tube is held tightly around the base of the penis to act as a tourniquet.

iii. The distal edge of the division of the skin lies one inch proximal to the lesion.

iv. A long dorsal or ventral skin flap is fashioned to cover the urethra.

v. The urethra with the corpus spongiosum is divided 2 cm distal to the corpora cavernosa to allow retraction.

vi. The corpora are vascular and require transfixion sutures of catgut.

vii. Releasing the tourniquet discloses vessels not under control.

viii. The urethra is brought out through an opening in the longer flap and a mucosa-to-skin approximation is carried out with catgut.

ix. Alternatively, the urethra is split and the two ends opened and held down by sutures, thereby reducing the risk of stricture.

x. A catheter may be left in for forty-eight hours.

126. TOTAL AMPUTATION OF PENIS AND BILATERAL ORCHIDECTOMY

i. Lithotomy position is used. The bladder is empty. A bougie is inserted into the urethra.

ii. A transverse incision across the symphisis is extended to encircle the scrotum and penis to terminate 2·5 cm from the anus in the midline.

iii. Depress the penis, expose, divide and ligate the dorsal vein and artery and divide the suspensory ligament.

iv. Elevate the penis, deepen the incision centrally, expose the bulb, then the penile urethra.

v. Mobilise the urethra and corpus spongiosum superficial to the triangular ligament and divide the urethra so that 1·5 cm are left to protrude outside the skin.

vi. Detach the corpora cavernosa from the ischiopubic ramus with a raspatory.

vii. Remove both testicles.

viii. Split and turn back the edges of the urethra to emerge at right angles to the triangular ligament. 1·5–2 cm should project beyond the wound. Alternatively, suture the edge of the urethra to the edge of the skin.

ix. Leave a catheter in for forty-eight hours.

127. HYPOSPADIAS

Denis Browne Operation

i. In the first stage (1–2 years) the penis is straightened by excising the fibroid "corpus spongiosum". Access is gained by a ventral transverse incision behind the glans. This is sewn up longitudinally.

ii. In the second stage (5–7 years), a perineal urethrostomy is established via the bulbous urethra.

iii. A strip of skin extending from the glans to a point beyond the urinary orifice is outlined by a knife and then buried by mobilising the skin on either side widely and suturing it together.

iv. The tension is relieved by a relieving incision made on the dorsum of the penis.

v. The dorsal wounds heal well because the penis never scars.

vi. The perineal urethrostomy tube is removed after ten days and the opening closes spontaneously, usually within a week.

128. DIVERTICULECTOMY

i. Open the bladder and, with stay sutures or tissue forceps, pull the mucosa of the diverticulum into the bladder; excise it and repair the hole in the vesical wall.

OR

ii. Open the bladder, infiltrate the wall with dilute adrenalin solution to reduce the bleeding. Cut around the neck of the diverticulum and dissect it out – keeping close to it. A catheter may be inserted into the ureter to help its identification.

OR

iii. Open the bladder, but approach the diverticulum from outside.

ALWAYS

iv. Drain the bladder continuously, per urethram or suprapubically, for seven days to avoid "blow-out" at the suture line and if necessary drain the extravesical cavity.

129. LITHOLAPAXY

i. Crushing of bladder stones by means of a special instrument (lithotrite) with a telescopic lens and light allows closure of blades to be seen, otherwise the instrument must be able to rotate freely before it is closed on the stone.

ii. 120 ml of fluid is left in the bladder, too much allows excessive movement of the stone. Too little endangers the bladder wall. The stones are engaged on the bladder base.

iii. Bigelow evacuator must be used with care to avoid bladder rupture. The stone fragments are washed out by it.

Contraindications to litholapaxy

i. A very large stone.

ii. A very hard or soft stone.

iii. A stone incorporating foreign body which is too large.

iv. A stone attached to the bladder wall or in a diverticulum.

v. A narrow urethra or bladder neck.

vi. A contracted bladder preventing adequate distension.

vii. A grossly diseased bladder.

viii. A patient below 10 years of age.

ix. A bladder containing a diverticulum.

x. Other pathology needing surgery.

130. HYDROCELE OPERATIONS

i. Approach is made through the scrotum if large, or via an inguinal incision. Inguinal approach must be used if it is thought that the hydrocele may be secondary to a diseased testis, thereby allowing high transection of cord.

ii. The sac is excised and its edges carefully ligated, or the sac is everted (Jaboulay) and sutured to maintain its position, or its wall plicated with a running suture (Lord).

131. STRICTURES OF THE URETHRA

Faced with obstruction due to an urethral stricture, urethrography is valuable.

i. Attempt to pass a small catheter, Tieman or a small Gibbon's catheter.
ii. If unsuccessful (with prostatic obstruction), coudé or bicoudé catheters are tried.
iii. If unsuccessful, try gum elastic bougies or whip-lash catheter, or employ "faggot" method with several fine bougies.
iv. If unsuccessful, perform external urethrotomy employing Wheelhouse staff and Teale's probe-pointed gorgette, or a suprapubic cystostomy.
v. Urethroscopy and division of stricture under vision may be attempted as an alternative.
vi. The stricture must be kept open by regular gentle dilatation.

Further Procedure for the Relief of Urethral Strictures

i. Excision with end-to-end (mucosa to mucosa) union of part or all of the circumference.
ii. Excision and invagination of the lower end of the urethra into the upper part (Badenoch).
iii. Restoring continuity with a strip of skin (Denis Browne).

132. RUPTURE OF MALE URETHRA

Five varieties

i. Extrapelvic – bulbar or penile.
ii. Intrapelvic, membranous urethra torn at the apex of the prostate.
iii. Partial or complete.
iv. With or without extravasation of urine.
v. With or without other injuries.

Five general principles in treatment

i. Avoid extravasation of urine by instructing the patient not to pass his water before he goes to operating theatre in suspected cases.

ii. Restore mucosal continuity as soon as possible employing one or two sutures.

iii. Avoid infection by draining any haematoma and preventing leakage of urine.

iv. Avoid strictures by leaving in catheters for prolonged period.

v. Urine is irritating, so bypass the flow, establish a suprapubic cystostomy, then carry out definitive repair after full investigations later.

Partial Injury of Bulbar Urethra

(Five points)

i. In Theatre, under sterile conditions, pass a soft rubber catheter.

ii. Cut down at the site of injury and leave it open to drain.

iii. Do not close the urethra.

iv. Leave in an indwelling catheter for four to five days.

v. Dilate the urethra after fourteen days and subsequently when necessary.

Complete Injury of Bulbar Urethra

(Five points)

i. Place patient in Lithotomy-Trendelenburg position.

ii. Open the bladder (and drain it subsequently through a suprapubic tube).

iii. Use a catheter to identify the urethra.

iv. Open the perineum at the site of the injury, restore continuity of the dorsal wall of the urethra with a few sutures of plain catgut, and leave in a small drain.

v. Dilate after two weeks and remove the suprapubic tube.

Complete Rupture of Membranous Urethra

(Five points)

i. Reduce a disrupted pelvic ring to assist approximation of the ends.

ii. If a catheter cannot be passed the patient is placed in the Lithotomy-Trendelenburg position so that the bladder may be opened and sounds passed via the urethra from above and below. The two ends of the urethra are aligned and a Foley catheter with its introducer is passed into the bladder.

iii. 900 g weight for 2 days and then 450 g weight for 10 days is applied to the catheter to approximate the ends.

iv. The urine is drained via a suprapubic tube which is removed after fourteen days.

v. The urethra is dilated subsequently as necessary.

Ruptured Urethra with Extravasation and Infection

i. Establish suprapubic drainage.

ii. Using multiple incisions drain the areas of extravasation.

iii. Drain any haematoma.

133. ORCHIDECTOMY

i. Patient's permission is obtained.

ii. Approach is the same as for inguinal hernia.

iii. The vas is separated from the cord. These structures are divided and ligated separately.

iv. A counter-incision in the scrotum may be necessary.

v. The conjoined tendon is sutured to the inguinal ligament to obliterate the internal ring.

vi. The external oblique, subcutaneous tissues and skin are closed.

134. EPIDIDYMECTOMY

i. General anaesthesia is employed. Permission to remove the testis, should this be necessary, is obtained.

ii. The operation is performed through an inguinal incision and if necessary a second scrotal incision is made.

iii. The vas is exposed as far as the internal ring. Its proximal end is carefully ligatured and dropped back, or it may be exteriorised if tuberculosis infection is present.

iv. The tunica vaginalis is opened and the epididymis and vas defined.

v. The epididymis is separated by a combination of sharp and blunt dissection from the testis, preserving the testicular artery and veins. Following the vas aids identification of the correct plane, and then both epididymis and vas are removed.

vi. Haemostasis is obtained and the wound closed.

135. ABDOMINAL HYSTERECTOMY (TOTAL)

i. The Trendelenburg position is used, the patient is catheterised and the vagina swabbed out with Bonney's blue.

ii. A midline or paramedian incision is made.

iii. Open the peritoneum and explore.

iv. Pack off the bowel and insert a self-retaining retractor.

v. Divide the round ligament, tube and a portion of the mesosalpinx on each side of the uterus between clamps.

vi. Open anterior leaf of broad ligament and extend mobilisation of it downwards to divide uterovesical fold of peritoneum.

vii. Mobilise the bladder from the uterus and upper part of the vagina by blunt dissection.

viii. The uterine vessels can be seen and are clamped, divided and ligated. Take care to avoid the ureters. The artery is anterior to the ureter.*

ix. The cardinal or Mackenrodt's ligaments are now clamped close to the uterus and divided, exposing the vaginal fornices.

x. The vaginal fornices are held and the circumference of the vagina divided.

xi. The vagina is closed completely, or left partly opened for drainage.

xii. The pelvic floor is re-peritonealised.

xiii. The packs are removed.

xiv The abdomen is closed.

CHAPTER XII

NEUROSURGERY

136. EXPOSURE OF THE BRAIN BY OSTEOPLASTIC FLAPS

i. General anaesthesia is used, e.g. hypophysectomy, or local anaesthesia in certain circumstances, e.g. coma, etc.

ii. According to circumstances, a sufficient area or the whole scalp is shaved, the skin incision lightly scratched with a knife.

iii. Moist gauze, usually soaked in 1:2000 Perchloride of Mercury, is then placed on the area, and the slight bleeding indicates the site for incision.

iv. The scalp is divided using the finger-tips to apply pressure to reduce bleeding, through the galea and pericranium, the former being grasped at 6 mm intervals with curved artery forceps which exert pressure and arrest the haemorrhage. These forceps are collected in bundles by elastic bands. A wide vascular base is necessary for all flaps.

v. The pericranium is reflected with a rugine.

vi. Burr-holes are cut with a Hudson's drill. Sufficient holes are made, varying with the size of flap.

vii. A Gigli saw is attached after an introducer has separated dura from bone. The bone is cut on a bevel to avoid subsequent "fall-in", Horsley's bone wax may aid haemostasis.

viii. The bone hinge is narrowed by bone-cutting forceps if the use of elevators fail to fracture it. The muscular hinge carries the blood supply.

ix. The dura is now exposed and bleeding vessels controlled with diathermy. The dura is elevated with a hook at a point clear of the cortical vessels, and divided with scalpel and dural scissors.

x. A surface tumour (meningioma) may be seen, deeper tumours may produce deformity of the convolutions or may be felt with a blunt ventricular needle.

xi. After closure with waxed silk threads the dura should be sutured to the pericranium or galea to prevent postoperative extradural haemorrhage. If an inoperable glioma is found, the skull flap is fixed to the skull with wire.

xii. Following the operation, the pericranium and galea are repaired with interrupted silk sutures.

xiii. The scalp is approximated on straight needles first, and sutures tied after the correct position has been achieved.

137. EXTRADURAL HAEMORRHAGE

i. The haematoma may lie in one of four areas – temporal, parietal, frontal, occipital.

ii. If local anaesthesia is used in an unconscious patient, intubation to ensure an adequate airway is essential.

iii. The scalp is shaved and prepared.

iv. The boggy scalp haematoma and the site of the skull fracture seen on the X-rays are the most reliable guides to the location of the extradural haematoma.

v. At the site of the suspected haemorrhage the scalp is incised down to the bone and a self-retaining retractor is inserted.

vi. The pericranium is stripped back with a rugine and a burr hole is made. If extradural clot is found the scalp wound is extended and the burr-hole is enlarged by nibbling away the bone with bone rongeurs until an opening large enough for the extraction of the clot has been made.

vii. Bleeding dural vessels are coagulated. Where the trunk of the middle meningeal artery is the source of the haemorrhage the vessel is transfixed and ligated or its bony canal is sealed with bone wax.

viii. Several burr-holes on both sides of the head may be necessary to locate the clot.

138. SUBDURAL HAEMATOMA

i. The haematoma is bilateral in 30 per cent of cases. Therefore the whole scalp is shaved.

ii. The patient is placed in the supine position with one side of the head rotated upwards.

iii. A frontal burr-hole, just within the hair line, and a posterior parietal burr-hole are made. The dura at both sites is opened. If liquid subdural blood is found it is aspirated and the subdural space is then gently irrigated with normal saline through a catheter.

iv. The wound is closed.

v. The head is rotated and the opposite subdural space is similarly explored.

vi. If the subdural blood is clotted, and this is often the case in acute subdural haematoma, an osteoplastic bone flap is made to facilitate the removal of the clot.

139. DIVISION OF TRIGEMINAL NERVE

i. Endotracheal anaesthesia is employed. The operation is performed with the patient seated.

ii. The approach is through the temporal fossa.

iii. An inverted hockey-stick incision is made just behind the half-way mark between the external angular process and the external auditory meatus. The "toe" of the hockey-stick points backwards. The incision terminates at the upper border of the zygoma. The lower part of the incision is curved backwards to avoid injury to the temporal branch of the facial nerve.

iv. A branch of the superficial temporal artery may require ligation and division.

v. The temporal fascia is divided, the muscle is split down to the infratemporal crest and a self-retaining retractor is inserted. An additional transverse cut through the fascia may be required. Approximately 13 cm^2 of the bone are exposed.

vi. The pericranium is divided and reflected.

vii. A burr-hole is made and enlarged with bone forceps.

viii. The base of the skull is exposed by elevating the dura upwards with the temporal lobe. A lighted retractor or head-light is employed.

ix. The middle meningeal vessels identified are followed to the foramen spinosum. Here they are divided after cauterisation by diathermy; immediately medial lies the mandibular branch. This is exposed and the visceral layer of dura mater divided and retracted a further 1·5 cm in an inward and backward direction to expose the sensory root posterior to the ganglion enclosed in its arachnoid sheath. This is opened. The motor root lies deeply, crosses posteriorly to the sensory fibres and is preserved.

x. If the neuralgia involves all of the distribution of the nerve, the whole sensory root is divided. If the symptom involves the second and third branches only, the outer two-thirds is divided.

xi. Following the division, absorbable cellulose haemostat may be applied to arrest ooze.

xii. The wound is closed in layers with silk.

140. VENTRICULAR TAPPING

Parietal Approach

i. Local anaesthesia is used. The head-end of the table is raised.

ii. Bilateral 2·5 cm long incisions are made 2·5 cm from the midline on the most prominent part of the parietal area, lying approximately 7·5 cm above the external occipital protuberance.

iii. The skin and galea are divided and the pericranium exposed by inserting a self-retaining retractor.

iv. The pericranium is divided and reflected to expose the bone.

v. A hole is then made with a perforator followed by a Hudson burr to expose the dura.

vi. Aim the cannula at the glabella to enter the ventricle approximately 4–5 cm from the dural surface.

vii. The galea and skin are approximated with interrupted silk sutures.

Frontal Approach

The burr-holes are made 2·5 cm from the midline just behind the hair line.

141. ASPIRATION OF BRAIN ABSCESS

i. A burr-hole is made at the appropriate site. Confirmation of the site may be made by arteriography, electroencephalography or the EMI scan. The wall of the abscess can often be felt by resistance against the ventricular cannula.

ii. The abscess is gently aspirated and pus sent for immediate microscopical examination and culture.

iii. 0·5 ml of microbarium sulphate is introduced so that the subsequent progress of the abscess may be observed radiographically. Antibiotic solution may also be introduced.

iv. Repeated aspiration over the subsequent days may be necessary.

v. Excision of the abscess may be carried out if the "capsule" is thick.

vi. In the case of a cerebellar abscess the first step is to tap the lateral ventricle through a posterior parietal burr-hole to relieve acute hydrocephalus. After this a suboccipital burr-hole is made and the abscess is aspirated.

142. TRANSFRONTAL APPROACH TO THE PITUITARY GLAND

i. An X-ray of the skull reveals the size of the frontal sinuses.

ii. General anaesthesia is employed.

iii. A right-sided approach is made through a small anterior osteoplastic flap based on the temporalis muscle.

iv. The dura is divided and the frontal lobe elevated, tracing the olfactory tract backward to reveal the optic nerve and then the chiasma; the pituitary lies behind this.

v. The diaphragm of the sella is incised in a cruciate manner. The stalk of the pituitary is defined. It runs almost horizontally backwards. This is clipped and divided. The pituitary is removed by pituitary rongeurs, sucker and gentle curette.

vi. The osteoplastic flap is returned and closed in layers.

143. COMPOUND FRACTURES OF SKULL

i. Ensure an adequate airway.

ii. The head-end of the table is raised to reduce venous congestion; foot-rest and knee-straps may be necessary.

iii. Local anaesthesia may be employed if unconscious.

iv. An intravenous drip is established. A Ryle's tube is in the stomach. Skull X-rays must be available in the theatre.

v. The scalp is shaved and prepared with antiseptic solution.

vi. The skin edges are excised and the wound extended. At this stage, pressure on the skin edges avoids blood loss from the scalp.

vii. Depressed areas of bone are raised directly or indirectly via a burr-hole or by raising an osteoplastic flap. The dura must be inspected for tears.

viii. Loose fragments of bone are best removed. Any fragments of bone in the brain must be removed. Damaged brain can be gently aspirated.

ix. Haemorrhage from the brain can be arrested by the use of diathermy or Cushing's silver (or tantalum) clips. Horsley's bonewax is used for bleeding bone.

x. Dural defects are made good by using fascia lata grafts obtained from the lateral aspect of the thigh or temporal muscle fascia.

xi. Fractured sinuses, such as the frontal sinus, are extensively explored, the contained mucosa is excised and the dura in the vicinity inspected and repaired with fascia if necessary, to avoid aerocele or rhinorrhoea with its danger of secondary infection.

144. POSTERIOR FOSSA APPROACH

Bilateral Exposure

i. The patient is placed in the sitting or the prone position, the head resting on a horseshoe-shaped support.

ii. An inverted U-shaped incision is made above or below the external occipital protuberance from behind the tip of one mastoid process to the other. Care is taken of the occipital artery. It is divided.

iii. The incision is deepened to expose the attachment of the spinal muscles to the superior nuchal line.

iv. The muscles are divided 6 mm below their attachments, leaving a fringe that may be used to restore them.

v. The muscle mass is stripped downwards to expose the occipital bone and the arch of the Atlas.

vi. Two burr-holes are made one on each side of the midline below the level of the transverse sinuses.*

vii. The openings are enlarged by nibbling the bone upwards as far as the transverse sinuses, laterally to the mastoid process but not opening the mastoid cells, and downwards to remove the posterior rim of the foramen magnum. Particular care must be taken to avoid opening emissary veins to prevent air embolism. The arch of Atlas may be removed. The dura is lifted up and incised, the inferior occipital sinus being clipped and divided.

viii. At the completion of the operation, the dura is repaired if possible.

ix. The spinal muscles are reconstituted with interrupted sutures.

Unilateral Exposure

i. A vertical midline incision is made midway between the midline and the mastoid process for midline lesions.

ii. An inverted hockey-stick incision is made for a lateral lesion.

145. DECOMPRESSION OF THE MEDIAN NERVE AT THE WRIST

i. A tourniquet is used.

ii. A median vertical incision 5 cm long is made over the palm, extending beyond the transverse crease of the wrist. Alternative incisions are transverse at the wrist, curved or shaped like a hockey-stick.

iii. The incision is deepened to expose the palmaris longus if present, and flexor carpi radialis. The median nerve lies between them in a deeper plane.

iv. The anterior carpal ligament is divided to decompress the nerve; this may be performed under vision, or the nerve protected and the division performed under the undivided skin.

v. The skin is sutured, a pressure dressing is applied and the tourniquet removed.

146. LAMINECTOMY AND CHORDOTOMY

i. General anaesthesia is used.

ii. The patient is placed in a sitting or prone position with the spine flexed, or prone with a sand-bag under the pelvis to avoid congestion of the spinal veins, and shoulder supports to facilitate respiration.

iii. A midline incision is made and skin towels applied.

iv. Deepen the incision to expose the spines.

v. Expose the spines and laminae by reflecting the erector spinae muscles with a wide raspatory.

vi. Insert a self-retaining muscle retractor.

vii. Remove spines at their base and the supra- and inter-spinous ligaments with bone-cutting forceps.

viii. Expose the dura by nibbling bone away from the laminae with bone forceps.

ix. Obtain haemostasis by using packs, bone-wax and ligatures.

x. Clear the dura of fat and coagulate veins.

xi. Pick up the dura with stay-sutures and open it for intradural lesions. Later re-suture it with silk.

xii. For chordotomy make a cut in the cord with a special angulated knife 3 mm deep from the denticulate ligament to the anterior nerve root on the appropriate side. (The fourth and fifth thoracic segments are opposite the second and third thoracic bodies.)

xiii. For removal of an intervertebral disc, perform a hemilaminectomy, remove one spinous process and retract the cord and nerve root. Divide the posterior longitudinal ligament over it, and curette it out with a pituitary rongeur.

xiv. Approximate the muscle and fascia with interrupted sutures.

xv. Close the skin.

147. THE MANAGEMENT OF THE PARAPLEGIC BLADDER (Guttmann)

i. During the first day the intake of fluids is restricted and attempts may be made to empty the bladder by manual compression.

ii. After this time, if unsuccessful, a medical officer empties the bladder eight hourly with a "non-touch" technique employing a small polythene catheter. The urine is tested repeatedly and antibiotics may be exhibited. In two to six weeks the automatic bladder may occur. This empties following cutaneous stimulation.

iii. With uncontrollable urinary infection an indwelling Foley catheter may be employed. The catheter is initially changed daily then extended to weekly intervals. The bladder is regularly washed out. Tidal drainage may be employed. Over-distension is carefully avoided but the bladder is allowed to fill and empty.

iv. In cauda equina lesions, emptying is performed by contracting the muscles of the anterior wall or by manual compression.

v. With the persistence of a high residual urine, bladder neck resections may be tried.

vi. Patients may be instructed to pass their own catheters and wash out their own bladders.

CHAPTER XIII

EAR AND EYE

148. Simple Mastoidectomy
149. Excision of Eyeball
150. Evisceration of Eye

148. SIMPLE MASTOIDECTOMY

i. General anaesthesia is used. An X-ray of the area is in Theatre.

ii. A curved incision is made, commencing at the upper attachment of the pinna and terminating below the mastoid tip. (The facial nerve lies subcutaneously in the infant.)

iii. The incision is deepended to the periosteum and a self-retaining retractor inserted.

iv. The periosteum is divided and reflected back to expose the mastoid process, and the superior and posterior borders of the bony meatus. The fibrocartilaginous meatus is not completely detached, to avoid meatal stenosis.

v. McEwen's triangle, the spine of Henle is present, and the direction of the bony meatus are used as guides in the exploration.

vi. The cortex of the mastoid process is removed with a broad gouge, including the outer wall of the tympanic antrum and other infected cells.

vii. The dura of the middle fossa and lateral sinus are seen and can be touched with a probe for identification – they feel soft.

viii. The skin is closed and the cavity drained.

149. EXCISION OF EYEBALL

i. General or local anaesthesia is employed.

ii. The conjunctiva is picked up close to the limbus, divided circumferentially and mobilised.

iii. Tenon's capsule is divided to expose the insertions of the rectus muscles, which are drawn forwards on a squint hook and divided at their insertions.

iv. Their tendons are doubly transfixed with linen sutures and the ends are left long.

v. A speculum is pressed posteriorly to protrude the eye and the oblique muscles and the optic nerve are divided. Scissors curved on the flat are used for dividing the nerve. Haemostasis is obtained by pressure from hot packs.

vi. An acrylic prosthesis may be used. This is held in by tying the rectus muscles about it in a cruciform pattern. This enables the prosthesis to move with the sound eye.

vii. If a prosthesis is not available, the muscle ends are tied together to form a knob which may function slightly.

viii. The conjunctiva is repaired with a running suture.

ix. A layer of tulle gras is applied.

x. The lids are closed and a built-up dressing applied.

150. EVISCERATION OF EYE

i. General anaesthesia is used.

ii. A circumferential incision is made in the periphery of the cornea, which is removed.

iii. The contents of the eyeball are removed.

iv. Haemostasis is secured with hot packs.

CHAPTER XIV

GENERAL ORTHOPAEDICS

151. Basic Principles for the Excision of a Compound Fracture
152. Important Orthopaedic Steps
153. Tendon Suture
154. Peripheral Nerve Suture with loss of nerve substance
155. Principles in Tendon Transplantation
156. Management of Traumatic Arterial Spasm
157. General Principles of Amputations
158. Above-Knee Myoplastic Flap
159. Through-Knee Amputation
160. Below-Knee Myoplastic
161. Below-Knee Amputation of Leg
162. Symes' Amputation
163. Fore-quarter Amputation
164. Hind-quarter Amputation
165. Disarticulation of the Shoulder
166. Excision of Shoulder Joint
167. Operation for Recurrent Dislocation of Shoulder
168. Excision of Elbow Joint
169. Excision of Head of Radius
170. Arthrodesis of Wrist Joint
171. Disarticulation of Hip
172. Arthrodesis of Hip Joint
173. Arthroplasty of Hip
174. Pinning of Femoral Neck
175. McMurray's Osteotomy
176. Excision of Knee Joint
177. Meniscectomy
178. Arthrodesis of Ankle Joint
179. Keller's Operation for Hallux Valgus
180. Mitchell's Operation for Hallux Valgus
181. Triple Arthrodesis of Foot

151. FIVE BASIC PRINCIPLES FOR THE EXCISION OF A COMPOUND FRACTURE

i. An extensive incision must be made so that the damaged areas may clearly be seen.

ii. Main arteries and nerves must be identified to avoid damage to them.

iii. Dead muscle, and damaged fascia skin and bone must be widely excised.

iv. The excision of these tissues is carried out before the bone is returned to its correct position.

v. Full thickness skin closure over bone must be maintained without tension, if necessary by use of a relief incision. Any deficiency over soft tissue is covered by a split skin graft.

152. FIVE IMPORTANT ORTHOPAEDIC STEPS

i. Apply pneumatic tourniquet after exsanguination noting the time of application and release. The application of it for one and a half hours is relatively safe.

ii. Employ a no-touch technique.

iii. Operate through steridrape to avoid skin contamination.

iv. On reaching bone, "stick close to it".

v. Apply pressure bandages before the removal of the tourniquet.

153. TENDON SUTURE

A primary tendon repair is performed in a clean incised wound, provided the tendon division does not lie between the distal palmar crease and the proximal finger crease. In all other cases complete skin healing, union of fractures and restoration of joint mobility must precede tendon repair.

i. A tourniquet is essential.

ii. The area of injury is explored and the distal cut end is mobilised. The discovery of the proximal end may require another incision placed at a higher level, in which case it is threaded through to the lower wound.

iii. The tendon ends are freshened and approximated with a Bunnell tendon suture, using steel wire or silk. When grafting, the palmaris longus the plantaris or the long extensors of the toes are used.

iv. Elevation of the limb avoids oedema.

v. Active movements follow three weeks after immobilisation.

154. PERIPHERAL NERVE SUTURE WITH LOSS OF NERVE SUBSTANCE

There are five ways of bridging the gap:

i. Extensive mobilisation by splitting up a branch to a higher level.

ii. Transposition, e.g. ulnar nerve.

iii. Partly flexing or extending a joint.

iv. Suturing in an autogenous graft: e.g. if two major nerves are damaged in the same injury and both are beyond suture, it may be possible to use a length of the less important nerve to bridge the gap in the more important one, either in one or two stages. A nerve graft should be 15 per cent "too long". The graft if large is inserted as a single trunk, if small it is built up as a "cable graft".

v. Employing a different nerve, e.g. accessory or hypoglossal to replace the proximal part of a facial nerve.

155. FIVE PRINCIPLES IN TENDON TRANSPLANTATION

i. The tendon transplant must be over a mobile joint. It will, of course, not correct a deformity.

ii. The tendon and muscle used must have sufficient strength to perform the task required of it.

iii. The alignment of the tendon should be as straight as possible from origin to its new insertion.

iv. Reattachment to bone is preferable to fixation of the tendon to other structures.

v. Immobilisation for three weeks is necessary, with additional protection for a further three weeks in the leg.

156. TRAUMATIC ARTERIAL SPASM

If conservative measures fail, such as fracture reduction, reflex heating, restoration of blood pressure, and the circulation does not return after one hour, expose the main artery at the site of injury and its branches through a long incision.

Where the vessel is found divided and adequate collateral circulation is present ligate both ends, if the collateral circulation is deemed inadequate remove clot freshen and suture the ends together, if impossible use a vein graft.

If the vessel is intact relieve spasm by the application of 2·5 per cent warm Papaverine solution. If spasm persists after fifteen minutes perform arteriotomy and proceed as for a divided vessel.

157. AMPUTATIONS

General principles

i. The use of tourniquets is avoided if the ischaemia is caused by arteriosclerosis.

ii. Equal anterior and posterior flaps are fashioned whenever feasible.

iii. Sites of election: In the upper arm, leave 20 cm, but if this is impossible, try to divide the bone 2·5 cm below the anterior axillary fold. Below the elbow, 17·5 cm of bone are preserved, but if this is impossible, the insertion of biceps should be preserved.
In the thigh, leave 25–28 cm, measured from trochanter tip, a length that leaves the insertion of adductor magnus. If this is not possible, at least 10 cm of bone are left as a minimum. Below the knee, leave 12·5 cm and a minimum of 5 cm, measured from the tibial tubercle.

iv. Points in the length of the stump:

(a) The joint above the prosthesis should flex without interference, and the stump should remain in its prosthesis.

(b) Muscles should be left to work the stump.

(c) The shorter the stump, the better the blood supply.

(d) Note, however, the longer the stump, the better the muscle control and leverage.

(e) Remove at least 7·5 cm above a joint to allow fitting of an artificial joint below it.

v. The deep fascia is dissected out with the skin and repaired as a separate layer, so that the skin can play over it. Main nerve endings are thereby separated from the moving skin.

vi. Muscles are divided at the line of bone section.

vii. Nerves: dissect the nerves upwards and cut them across with a sharp knife. They should not be ligated.

viii. The main vessels are doubly ligated with non-absorbable ligatures. It is customary to transfix the distal ligature as an additional safeguard. The bone is divided carefully, leaving no spurs. The periosteum is divided with a knife and deflected downwards to allow for the siting of the saw. Sharp subcutaneous edges are bevelled to avoid subsequent damage to the flaps.

ix. Haemostasis is obtained and the flaps are brought together loosely in the leg.

x. Drainage tubes are left in for twenty-four hours. Following the removal of the drains, the openings may be closed by applying Michel clips.

xi. In children, above the knee and below the elbow amputations should be constructed to leave an ample soft tissue margin to allow for bone growth.

158. ABOVE-KNEE MYOPLASTIC FLAP

i. The patient lies supine. Mark the leg at the site of election. The diameter of limb is equal to half of the circumference which can be measured by tape, thus giving the length of flap from the site of election.

ii. Fashion equal anterior and posterior flaps including the deep fascia and reflect them to a point 2·5 cm above proposed line of bone section.

iii. Mark the muscle groups, arbitrarily divided into four quadrants, by four stay sutures at level of proposed bone section.

iv. Divide the muscles 2·5 cm shorter than the skin flaps and reflect them to level of bone section.

v. Divide main vessels and nerves.

vi. Reflect area of periosteum (if possible) to cover raw area of bone, retract soft tissues, divide bone, shave off any sharp edge and cover it, with the periosteum.

vii. Check on haemostasis.

viii. Cover the bone end by suturing over it in turn the lateral then the anterior and posterior muscle groups, opposing groups being sutured to each other.

ix. Resuture the deep fascia, subcutaneous tissues.

x. Close skin providing two lateral drains.

xi. Care flexion deformity developing at level of the hip joint, employ physiotherapy and splintage.

159. THROUGH-KNEE AMPUTATION

The condyles of the femur provide a good weight bearing platform.

i. Cut a square-ended skin flap from the medial to the lateral hamstring tendons extending down to a level 7·5 cm below the tibial tubercle with the knee flexed. The base of the flap should be more than half the leg's circumference. The posterior flap is made and extends 5 cm below the joint with the knee extended. Divide patella tendon and reflect it with skin integument.

ii. Flex the knee joint open excise the synovia and menisci. Divide the capsule and cruciate ligaments, leaving the latter long.

iii. Extend the knee and divide gastrocnemius and ham strings.

iv. Divide vessels and nerves.

v. Suture patella tendon and hamstrings to the cruciate ligaments.

vi. Trim skin flaps to provide posterior suture line.

160. MYOPLASTIC TECHNIQUE OF BELOW-KNEE AMPUTATION (BURGESS)

i. Patient is placed in the supine position.

ii. Make an incision across the front of the leg 12·5 cm below the knee joint.

iii. Deepen the incision down to the tibia.

iv. Reflect proximally the anterior tibial muscles and periosteum for 1·25 cm.

v. Divide and bevel the tibia. Dissect it out and divide the fibula 2·5 cm above this level.

vi. Extend the ends of the skin incision vertically downwards for 15 cm and connect them together posteriorly thus constituting the posterior flap. Reflect this flap upwards. Find the sural nerve and divide it clear of the site of the election.

vii. Deepen the posterior incision through the muscles down to the tibia and fibula, reflect them upwards and remove the leg.

viii. Model muscles and then suture them over the site of bone division.

ix. Achieve haemostasis.

x. Close muscle, fascia and skin with drainage.

161. BELOW-KNEE AMPUTATION OF LEG

i. The patient lies in the supine position towards the end of the table. The affected leg is held by an assistant beyond the table, and the sound leg is allowed to flex at the knee, and is supported on a stool and between sand-bags. The skin is prepared and towels are applied.

ii. The site of election is 12·5 cm below the tibial tubercle. Equal anterior and posterior flaps are cut below this level. The length of each flap is half the diameter of the limb.

iii. The skin flaps are reflected with the deep fascia, the muscles are divided down to the bone, the fibula is dissected free and divided 3·8 cm above the site* chosen for the tibia.

iv. The periosteum is then cut through with a knife and the tibia divided with a saw at right angles to the bone. The anterior edge of the tibia is cut away to produce a bevelled effect.

v. The main vessels are doubly ligated and if a tourniquet is present, it is released to obtain final haemostasis.

vi. The skin is closed, and the wound is drained.

162. SYMES' AMPUTATION

i. General anaesthesia is used. A tourniquet may be applied.

ii. The foot is held at right angles over the end of the table.

iii. Hold the malleoli and make an incision from the lateral malleolar tip vertically down to the sole, cross is transversely, continue it over the medial aspect of the ankle terminating 12 mm below the medial malleolar tip. If taken 12 mm behind the medial malleolus, the calcaneal branch of the lateral plantar artery may be damaged.*

iv. Dissect off the heel flap by keeping close to the bone. Laterally, the flap is supplied by the terminal branches of the peroneal artery.

v. Divide the Achilles tendon.

vi. Depress the foot and incise across the dorsum through the tendons and down to the bone.

vii. Disarticulate by dividing the ligaments – the lateral ligament from within outwards.

viii. Catch the vessels and ligate them.

ix. Retract the soft tissues and remove the malleoli and tibial articular cartilage by sawing across the bone as low as possible. Avoid removing the epiphysis in the young.

x. Release tourniquet, obtain haemostasis, leave in drain and sew up.

xi. An "elephant boot" is used when the parts are soundly healed.

163. FORE-QUARTER AMPUTATION

i. The patient lies supine with the affected shoulder overhanging the table-edge with an assistant holding the arm.

ii. The subclavian vessels and brachial plexus are exposed by excising the middle third of the clavicle through an incision made above it.

iii. The vessels and nerves are divided.

iv. The lateral end of the incision is extended downwards across the anterior axillary fold to reach the inferior angle of the scapula.

v. The incision is deepened to expose and divide the pectoral muscles.

vi. The arm is then adducted and the remaining part of the "raquet"-shaped incision is carried vertically downwards over the scapula.

vii. The skin of the back is then raised to expose the medial edge of the scapula and its attached muscles are divided.

viii. Haemostasis if obtained and the wound sutured, leaving in drain.

164. HIND-QUARTER AMPUTATION

i. An assistant holds the limb to be removed and the patient is tilted partly over on to his sound side to expose the posterior superior iliac spine.

ii. The incision commences behind the posterior superior iliac spine, runs along the iliac crest to a point 5 cm below and medial to the anterior superior iliac spine, then parallel to the inguinal ligament to a point 3·8 cm below the pubic spine.

iii. The incision is deepened to expose the anterior abdominal wall muscles. The muscles are divided to expose the external iliac vessels and the peritoneum.

iv. The main vessels are ligated immediately above the inguinal ligament.

v. The spermatic cord is mobilised and drawn upwards and medially.

vi. The inguinal ligament is detached at each end.

vii. All aspects of the symphisis pubis are cleared and it is divided with a Gigli saw.

viii. The patient is tilted further over on to the sound side.

ix. The incision is extended by cutting vertically down from the middle point of the iliac crest as far as the gluteal fold, continued in this fold to the medial aspect of the thigh running forwards to meet the termination of the original incision.

x. The skin flaps are raised, the glutei divided to expose the dorsum ilii leaving a fringe of gluteus maximus posteriorly.

xi. The pelvis is divided through the greater sciatic notch.

xii. The lumbosacral trunk, the first and second sacral nerves, the obturator nerve, are divided.

xiii. The obturator, gluteal, sciatic and internal pudendal vessels, are divided and ligated.

xiv. The psoas, piriformis, levator ani, ischiocavernosus and crus penis are divided.

xv. The limb is removed.

xvi. The end is covered by suturing together the abdominal muscles to the levator ani and gluteus maximus.

xvii. The skin is approximated and the wound drained.

165. DISARTICULATION OF THE SHOULDER

i. The patient is placed close to the table edge, the arm is abducted and externally rotated.

ii. The incision commences lateral to the coracoid, extends down the arm to the lateral extremity of the anterior axillary fold, around the arm to level of the posterior fold, and over the medial aspect of the arm to meet the vertical part of the incision.

iii. Deepen the anterior part of the incision. Expose and mobilise pectoralis major and divide it.

iv. Retract the pectoral muscle exposing the axillary vessels, and ligate them; artery first, elevate the arm, then tie the vein.

v. Divide the deltoid down to the bone and reflect this muscle upwards.

vi. Rotate the arm medially and detach supraspinatus, infraspinatus and teres minor.

vii. Divide the anterior part of joint capsule and the long head of biceps.

viii. Rotate the arm laterally and divide the subscapularis.

ix. Further abduct the arm, and dislocate the head.

x. Hold the head outwards and divide the posterior capsule, the long head of triceps, the teres major, the latissimus dorsi, the short head of biceps and coracobrachialis.

xi. Keep close to bone. Take care of circumflex arteries.

xii. Divide the structures on the medial side of arm by a sweep of the knife.

xiii. Section the nerves clear of the wound.

xiv. Check the ligatures on the main vessels and use a transflxion stitch distally.

xv. Excise the synovia. Attend to haemostasis.

xvi. Suture the skin and drain.

166. EXCISION OF THE SHOULDER JOINT

i. The patient lies supine with the arm slightly abducted. The coracoid process is thrown into prominence by a sand-bag placed under the angle of the scapula.

ii. An incision is made 15 cm long from the coracoid process downwards one finger breadth lateral to deltopectoral groove.

iii. The head of the bone and the long head of biceps is exposed by splitting the deltoid in line of the incision and retracting the edges of the muscle. This step avoids the cephalic vein.

iv. The long head of the biceps is dissected off, retracted and preserved.

v. The arm is rotated medially and with a periosteal elevator the muscles attached to the greater tuberosity of the humerus are detached.

vi. The arm is rotated laterally and the subscapularis is similarly stripped off from the lesser tuberosity.

vii. The capsule is picked up and divided, the head of the humerus is dislocated by pushing the arm upwards and backwards.

viii. The head of the humerus is cleared of muscles and divided with a saw. The inner edge of the bone is bevelled so that it is less likely to damage the neurovascular bundle.

ix. Further excision of the capsule or glenoid labrum may be necessary.

x. Haemostasis is obtained, a stab drain is inserted emerging posteriorly.

xi. The skin is closed.

167. OPERATION FOR RECURRENT DISLOCATION OF SHOULDER (Bankhart)

The humeral head may be thrust forwards, tearing off the fibrocartilaginous labrum glenoidale. This structure fails to re-attach itself, but simple capsular tears will undergo spontaneous repair.

A defect of the humeral head may be present.

i. A sand-bag is placed between the scapulae to allow the shoulder to fall backwards. The incision commences above the coracoid process, extends downwards one finger-breadth lateral to the deltopectoral groove for 12·5 cm.

ii. Identify and preserve the cephalic vein.

iii. Divide the deep fascia and split the deltoid in line with the incision.

iv. If exposure is inadequate identify and divide the coracoid process; retract the tip and its attached muscles downwards.

v. Rotate the arm laterally and divide the subscapularis after inserting stay-sutures and also the capsule 2·5 cm from the muscle insertion.

vi. Open and inspect the capsule, and retract the humeral head with Bankhart's retractor.

vii. If the lesion is present, that is, the labrum is detached or split, raise a shaving from the front of the glenoid cavity to produce a raw area.

viii. Drill holes in the anterior edge of the glenoid with an angled dental drill.

ix. Suture the detached glenoidal labrum to the raw area, using wire, nylon or other suitable ligatures.

x. Repair the subscapularis (in the Putti-Platt operation the muscle and capsule are overlapped for 2·5 cm).

xi. Resuture the coracoid process into position, if divided.

xii. Bandage the arm to the side with the elbow held forwards for five weeks. This ensures that the humeral head is held at the back of the joint.

168. EXCISION OF ELBOW JOINT

i. Apply a tourniquet.

ii. Place the arm at 30 degrees short of full extension.

iii. Commence the incision at a point three finger-breadths above the lateral epicondyle, down over supracondylar ridge across the lateral aspect of joint, over the head of radius along the lateral border of anconeus to a point on the posterior border of the ulna.

iv. Deepen the incision to bone, separate off the common extensor origin and the brachioradialis, then deepen the incision through the ligaments embracing the head of the radius.

v. Keep close to the bone and raise the triceps, posterior part of capsule, triceps insertion and anconeus to expose the posterior aspects of the joint. Extending the arm helps this mobilisation. Clear the medial epicondyle and front of joint, preserving the brachialis and biceps.* Excise the joint.

169. EXCISION OF HEAD OF RADIUS

i. The head and the neck of the radius is exposed by an incision made over it commencing above the lateral epicondyle, or from the lateral epicondyle to the ulna along the lateral border of the anconeus.

ii. The head is exposed by dissecting between the extensor carpi ulnaris and the extensor digitorum communis.

iii. By keeping close to the bone,* damage to the posterior interosseous nerve is avoided.

iv. The periosteum and capsule are divided and the bone cut with an osteotome proximal or distal to the annular ligament.

v. Meticulous removal of fragments of bone, periosteum and capsule is carried out to avoid ankylosis.

vi. The soft tissues above the cut end of bone are sutured over it.

vii. Haemostasis obtained, the wound is closed.

viii. The arm is held at a right-angle for ten days.

ix. Removal of the head of the radius must not be done in children because of the gross deformity that results.*

170. ARTHRODESIS OF WRIST JOINT

i. A vertical incision is made over the posterior aspect of the wrist joint in line with the third metacarpal bone.

ii. The tendons are retracted to expose the joint surface.

iii. The articular surfaces of the carpus and the lower end of the radius are excised and the cavities filled with bone chips obtained from the ilium, supplemented by a cortical graft from the ulna.

iv. Excising the lower 5 cm of the ulna maintains pronation and supination.

v. The skin is closed, the wrist and forearm are put in plaster for fourteen weeks with slight dorsiflexion at the wrist.

171. DISARTICULATION OF HIP

i. The incision runs parallel and 5 cm below the inguinal ligament.

ii. The deep fascia is divided to expose the femoral vessels.

iii. The femoral vessels are dissected free, doubly ligated and divided.

iv. The muscles are divided down to the hip joint.

v. The joint capsule is divided and the femoral head dislocated and freed.

vi. The thigh is raised and the posterior flap made equal to the diameter of the limb (one-third of the measured circumference of the limb).

vii. The posterior flap is reflected to expose the ischium and the muscles and nerves are divided close to the pelvis.

viii. Haemostasis is obtained, the skin flaps closed and the wound drained.

172. INTRA-ARTICULAR ARTHRODESIS OF HIP

i. Five prerequisites for the arthrodesis:

(a) The lumbar spine should be mobile.

(b) There should be good knee movements on both sides.

(c) There should be good hip movements on the other side.

(d) The patient should be young.

(e) It should not be done for tuberculosis.

ii. Expose the hip joint using the lateral approach. A vertical incision is drawn over the greater trochanter.

iii. The incision is deepened through the fascia lata separating the gluteus maximus from the fascia lata.

iv. The muscles are separated from the greater trochanter and the capsule exposed and opened.

v. The femoral head is dislocated from the acetabulum by flexing the femur and rotating it medially.

vi. The joint surfaces are removed until cancellous bone is exposed.

vii. Fixation is achieved by inserting a trifin nail through the femoral neck into the bone above the acetabulum. Bone chips are added.

viii. Any deformity is corrected before the nail is introduced or by performing a subtrochanteric osteotomy. The wounds are closed.

ix. A skeletal traction pin is inserted through the tibial tubercle and weight is applied to maintain the correct position for six weeks, after which a short plaster spica is applied (Pyrford).

173. APPROACHES TO AND ARTHROPLASTIES OF HIP

A. Anterior Smith-Petersen approach

i. Improve access by rotating patient to the opposite side and placing a sandbag under the sacrum, supero-medial to the sciatic nerve, and another under the shoulder blade.

ii. The incision runs along the iliac crest to the anterior-superior iliac spine, then passes downwards between the sartorius and the tensor fascia lata.

iii. The sartorius and the anterior portion of the Glutius Medius are mobilised from the ilium.

iv. The capsule is now exposed and divided just lateral to the lower acetabulum, thence up to the top of the femoral neck and continued laterally to the greater trochanter. The reflected head of the rectus is divided with the capsule and retracted medially.

Points in Arthroplasty

Any of the approaches to the hip joint described may be used.
Thompson or Lustrelite prostheses may be employed for intracapsular fractures of the femoral neck.
The exposed femoral head is removed by a cork-screw like instrument and bone levers.
The femoral neck is trimmed with an osteotome.
Ream the femur. Insert the cement and prosthesis.
Reduce the prosthesis.
Close wound in layers include a suction drain.

Replacement Arthroplasties

i. Lateral or posterior approaches may be used. The Greater Trochanter is removed in the Charnley operation.

ii. The head is dislocated and then excised by power saw or osteotome.

iii. The acetabulum is reamed.

iv. The centering hole is closed by a mesh cup in the Charnley operation. The cement is inserted followed by the acetabular component.

v. The femoral shaft is reamed. The cement and prosthesis are inserted.

vi. The femoral prosthesis is reduced.

vii. The trochanter, is divided, is replaced and fixed with wire sutures.

viii. The wound is closed in layers and a suction drain included.

B. Posterior approach of Gibson

i. The patient lies on the unaffected side with the upper arm on a rest, and the chest and back supported by padded rests.

ii. The skin is incised along the anterior border of the gluteus maxims to the greater trochanter and then downwards for 15 cm approximately.

iii. The iliotibial band is incised in line with the lower limb of the incision, and the gluteal bursa opened.

iv. The gluteus maximus is then separated and retracted medially.

v. The gluteus medius and minimus are now freed and retracted.

vi. The capsule is then exposed by retracting the quadratus femoris, and dividing the piriformis with the gemelli.

vii. The capsule is opened in T-shaped manner and the hip dislocated by rotating the thigh medially.

viii. (a) A Thompson prosthesis may be inserted.
Stages as under the anterior approach.

(b) McKee Hip Replacement.

1. Femoral head dislocated and removed.
2. Acetabulum reamed and drilled for cement.
3. Acetabular prosthesis located.
4. Femoral prosthesis inserted as in viii (*a*).

ix. Wound closed in layers with "haemovac" drainage.

174. INTERNAL FIXATION BY A SMITH-PETERSEN PIN

i. An orthopaedic table is used.

ii. The fracture is reduced by traction in flexion and followed by internal rotation and abduction.

iii. This position is maintained and the X-ray apparatus is set up.

iv. X-rays of the hip are used in two planes to ensure satisfactory reduction. An image intensifier may be used.

v. Through a 10 cm lateral incision the trochanter and the upper part of the femur is exposed.

vi. To facilitate the introduction of the guide wire, a circular disc of cortex is removed from an area 12 mm below the great trochanter.

vii. Guide wires are inserted until the correct position of one of them is achieved, confirmed by radiograph, and the required length of nail estimated.

viii. The canalised trifin type of nail is then driven over the guide wire into the head. The wire is removed and the fracture is impacted. The position of the nail is checked by further X-rays.

ix. In the case of intertrochanteric fractures further fixation is obtained by a plate that holds the end of the nail and can be screwed down into the lateral aspect of the shaft of femur.

x. The wound is closed.

xi. Movements are commenced on the day after operation.

175. OSTEOTOMY OF FEMUR (McMurray)

i. Under the anaesthesia the degree of fixed deformity is confirmed. The patient is placed on the orthopaedic table in this position. The femur is exposed through a lateral incision.

ii. The shaft is divided upwards and inwards below the lesser trochanter so that the proximal end of the distal fragment may be displaced inwards by half the diameter of the femur. The weight-bearing line is thereby altered and the existing deformity may be corrected.

iii. Fixation is achieved by a nail plate or a spline. In the former technique the nail is inserted prior to the osteotomy. Bony union is achieved in three to four months.

176. EXCISION OF KNEE JOINT WITH ARTHRODESIS

i. A tourniquet may be employed.

ii. The operation is performed with the knee flexed over the end of the table, or with the knee extended.

iii. A U-shaped incision is made with the lower part crossing the tibial tubercle.

iv. The skin is reflected upwards to expose the patellar tendon, which is detached together with the lateral aspects of the knee joint capsule. This exposes the joint and its contents.

v. The cartilage overlying the bones is removed and the saw cuts so made to allow the tibia and femur to come together in a good position, correcting any pre-existing deformity.

vi. Further fixation may be established by using crossed pins, a tibial inlay, or bedding down the "rawed" patella. Alternatively, skeletal pins are passed through each bone and compressed together with an external screw device (Charnley). The deep fascia is sutured, and the skin closed, and the leg encased in plaster with five degrees of flexion to avoid genu recurvatum.

177. MENISCECTOMY

i. Exsanguinate with an Esmarch tourniquet and maintain it with a pneumatic tourniquet. The thigh is supported on a sand-bag.

ii. The skin is prepared.

iii. The knee is flexed over the end of the table.

iv. An incision 4 cm long commences 2·5 cm above the joint level at the anterior edge of the medial ligament and passes over the joint line downwards and outwards to the medial edge of the patellar ligament. This incision avoids the infrapatellar branch of the saphenous nerve.

v. Employing another scalpel, the capsule is divided in line with the incision.

vi. The synovium is incised superiorly to prevent suction of it against the femoral condyles. The cartilage and other joint structures are inspected.

vii. The medial collateral ligament is then retracted to obtain a view of the peripheral attachment of the cartilage.

viii. The anterior horn of the meniscus is then detached, using a scalpel.

ix. The cartilage is firmly held in the left hand with a cartilage clamp and drawn inwards towards the intercondylar space, dividing the peripheral attachment with a solid scalpel.

x. The posterior horn is then divided, taking care to avoid injuring the posterior cruciate ligament.* Rotation of the tibia laterally and flexion of the knee may help in this division. This is best achieved by keeping the knife stationary and drawing the cartilage over it.

xi. The synovia and capsule are sutured separately. The skin is closed.

xii. A pressure bandage is applied.

xiii. The tourniquet is removed.

Excision of the Posterior End of the Medial Cartilage

A vertical 5 cm incision may be made behind and parallel with the medial ligament to remove the posterior end of the medial cartilage.

178. ARTHRODESIS OF ANKLE JOINT

i. The ankle is fixed in five degrees of equinus to allow for the standing position wearing a heel. It is neither inverted or everted.

ii. The joint is approached anteriorly by employing a 12 cm incision made over the tibialis anterior tendon.

iii. The tendon, vessels and nerves are retracted to expose the anterior surface of the joint.

iv. The joint is opened and the opposing cartilaginous surfaces are removed.

v. The position may be stabilised by cutting a slightly tapered graft from the front of the tibia, turning it upside down and fixing it into the tibial trench above and in a prepared socket in the talus below (Watson Jones), or using Charnley's compression clamp.

vi. The leg and foot are encased in a plaster of Paris cast.

179. KELLER'S OPERATION FOR HALLUX VALGUS

i. A tourniquet is applied.

ii. An incision is made over the anteromedial aspect of the proximal phalanx and metatarsophalangeal joint of the big toe.

iii. The joint is opened medial to the extensor hallucis longus tendon.

iv. The proximal third of the proximal phalanx is excised, preserving the flexor hallucis longus tendon.

v. The exostosis of the metatarsal head is excised.

vi. The skin is closed.

vii. A pad of gauze between the toes maintains the varus position.

viii. Following operation, early movements are initiated.

180. MITCHELL'S OPERATION FOR HALLUX VALGUS

i. A tourniquet is applied.

ii. An incision is made over the anteromedial aspect of the distal half of the first metatarsal to just beyond the metatarsal joint.

iii. Elevate the capsule on the medial side by means of triangular flap of soft tissue (apex based proximally) exposing the exostosis on the metatarsophalangeal joint.

iv. The exostosis is removed with an osteotome.

v. The first metatarsal bone is drilled at two points, the distal hole being more medial so that after displacing the distal portion laterally the two holes are brought in line.

vi. The first metatarsal is divided obliquely at its distal one third so that it can be impacted on to the proximal spike.

vii. A suture is passed through the drill holes and tied to increase stability.

viii. The subluxation of the metatarsophalyngeal joint is reduced by suturing the soft tissue flap to the proximal periosteum and after skin closure this position is maintained by wooden spatulae employed as splints.

ix. Ten days later a below-knee P.O.P. including the Great Toe is applied and maintained with weight bearing until X-ray evidence of union is seen, approximately 6 to 8 weeks.

181. TRIPLE ARTHRODESIS OF FOOT
(Naughton Dunn)

i. Arthrodeses are established between the calcaneum and cuboid, talus and cuneiforms, and talus and calcaneum. The navicular is removed.

ii. The incision commences 7·5 cm above the lower end of the fibula, curves round below it, crosses the dorsum of the foot to terminate opposite the third metatarsal bone.

iii. The peroneal tendons are displaced or alternatively divided and resutured at the end of the operation.

iv. The joint surfaces between the calcaneum and cuboid are first removed.

v. The structures covering the joints medially are mobilised and retracted.

vi. The joints are opened and the navicular is excised together with the cartilaginous surfaces of the head of the talus and cuneiforms.

vii. The subtalar joint is opened after dividing the interosseous talocalcaneal and the calcaneofibular ligament.

viii. The foot is dislocated medially and the opposed cartilages of the subtalar joint removed.

ix. More bone is removed from the medial portion of the foot for a valgus deformity and the lateral part for the varus deformity.

x. The raw ends of the bones are brought together and the foot moulded in a plaster cast.

CHAPTER XV

BLOOD VESSELS

182. General Principles of Arterial Operations
183. Trendelenburg Operation
184. Ligation of Incompetent Perforators of the Leg
185. Ligation of Common Carotid
186. Ligation of External Carotid
187. Carotid Endarterectomy
188. Ligation of Third Part of Subclavian Artery
189. Exposure of Innominate Artery
190. Exposure of Brachial Artery
191. Exposure of Terminal Part of Brachial Artery
192. Exposure of External Iliac Artery
193. Exposure of Femoral Artery upper two thirds
194. Exposure of Popliteal Artery
195. Exposure of the Posterior Tibial and Peroneal Arteries
196. Femoropopliteal Arterial Bypass with Reversed Vein
197. Extraction of Saddle-embolus
198. Graft Replacement of Abdominal Aortic Aneurysm
199. Micro-vascular Surgery – Digital Reimplantation
200. Inferior Vena Cava Ligation

182. GENERAL PRINCIPLES OF ARTERIAL OPERATIONS

i. Incisions should follow the course of arteries to allow their extension.

ii. Dissection is kept close to the artery. Tapes passed round an artery help to elevate it and facilitate clamp application.

iii. Proximal and distal control is necessary.

iv. Branches are preserved but may be temporarily occluded with a double loop of thick silk held in an artery forceps.

v. Intravenous heparin is given 5 minutes before clamp application except in cases of trauma and haemorrhage. Its action may be reversed with protamine sulphate.

vi. Non-absorbable, double-ended sutures are used. Whenever possible the needle should enter through the intima and emerge from the adventitia.

vii. Endarterectomy. The artery is incised longitudinally and the occluding plug is dissected out. The distal cut edge of intima is sutured to the adventitia. A patch graft may be sutured into the arteriotomy to avoid narrowing the arterial lumen.

viii. Grafts. These are synthetic (Dacron, Teflon) or autogenous (Long saphenous or cephalic vein). Extensive aorto-iliac occlusive disease is treated with an aortofemoral Dacron bifurcated bypass graft. Vein is preferred for bypass grafting in the extremities.

ix. Aneurysms. These are excluded from the circulation by proximal and distal ligation or they are excised. Blood flow is restored with a bypass graft or a replacement graft.

183. TRENDELENBURG AND STRIPPING OF LONG SAPHENOUS VEIN

i. An incision is made below and parallel with the inguinal ligament. It overlies the femoral pulse and the middle of the incision is a finger-breadth below and lateral to the pubic spine.

ii. The incision is deepened to expose the saphenous vein.

iii. The saphenous vein and its tributaries are dissected free of the surrounding structures until a clear view is obtained of the junction of the vein with the femoral vein.

iv. The various tributaries are divided.

v. The saphenous vein is then doubly ligated and divided close to its junction.

vi. An incision is now made over the long saphenous vein in front of the medial malleolus, and the vein is mobilised.

vii. An incision is made into it, and a stripper is introduced.

viii. The distal end of the vein is divided and ligated. The vein is securely tied to the stripper just proximal to its head.

ix. The small wound is now closed. The inguinal incision is partly closed.

x. The vein is now stripped out from below upwards.

xi. During the stripping, the leg is bandaged from below upwards to reduce subcutaneous oozing.

xii. The remaining part of the inguinal incision is closed.

184. LIGATION OF INCOMPETENT PERFORATING VEINS OF LEG
(Cockett)

i. The patient lies supine with the legs partially abducted. The Trendelenburg tilt reduces the venous engorgement.

ii. For the medial perforators an incision is made one finger-breadth behind the medial margin of the tibia in the lower half of the leg. It does not extend beyond the medial malleolus. For the vessels on the lateral side a vertical incision is made along the lateral aspect of the lower part of the leg. Either incision may run through the ulcer or the ulcer may be excised and the raw area grafted at the end of the operation.

iii. The dissection is deepened to expose the deep fascia and the dissection continues on this plane until the vessels are discovered. They are then ligated and divided.

iv. The usual sites for the vessels are just above the medial malleolus, four fingers-breadth above the medial malleolus, and at the midpoint of the leg.

v. If the perforators are not discovered superficial to the deep fascia (as suggested by Cockett) the fascia is divided and the vessels are sought deep to it.

vi. The skin is sutured only.

vii. A Trendelenburg operation with stripping of the saphenous vein is performed.

viii. The leg is bandaged with a web elastic bandage, the patient returned to the ward and the leg is elevated for two days.

185. COMMON CAROTID LIGATION

i. Local anaesthesia is used, the effect of a 20-minute ligation can thus be assessed.*

ii. A skin crease incision is made at the level of the cricoid cartilage.

iii. The incision is deepened through the platysma to expose the anterior margin of the sternomastoid.

iv. The external jugular vein may require division.

v. The anterior margin of sternomastoid is mobilised to expose the carotid sheath, the decendens hypoglossi and the anterior belly of the omohyoid.

vi. The thyroid veins require ligation.

vii. The artery is dissected free. An aneurysm needle is passed away from the vein, and the artery ligated.

viii. Note: If the artery is ligated and *divided* the vasoconstrictor nerves are similarly interrupted, a clot formed above the ligature is less easily dislodged as a distal embolus, and bleeding is less likely to occur. The divided vessel end contracts, and recanalisation cannot occur.

186. EXTERNAL CAROTID LIGATION

i. Local or general anaesthesia is used.

ii. A skin crease incision is made 2·5 cm below the angle of the jaw to avoid the cervical branch of the facial nerve.

iii. The incision is deepened through the platysma to expose the external jugular and common facial veins.

iv. The anterior margin of the sternomastoid is defined and the muscle mobilised.

v. The lingual vein is divided and the posterior belly of the digastric retracted upwards to expose the artery.

vi. The hypoglossal nerve is seen and preserved.

vii. The pulsation of the artery is felt* and its branches are seen.* The internal carotid lies deep to it.

viii. The artery is ligated.

187. CAROTID ENDARTERECTOMY

i. The head is extended and turned to the opposite side.

ii. An incision is made along the anterior border of the sternomastoid muscle.

iii. The deep fascia is divided in the line of the incision and the sternomastoid is retracted backwards.

iv. The common, external and internal carotid arteries are dissected free and overlying veins divided. The hypoglossal nerve crossing superficial to the external and internal carotid arteries is identified and preserved.

v. Intravenous heparin is given.

vi. The stenotic proximal segment of the internal carotid artery is gently palpated and the vessel is clamped beyond this.

vii. The common and external carotid arteries are clamped.

viii. Endarterectomy is performed.

ix. The arteriotomy is carefully closed to avoid narrowing the vessel or a Teflon patch is sutured in place.

x. The clamps on the external, common and internal carotid arteries are removed.

xi. Protamine is injected intravenously to reverse the action of the heparin.

(Note: To maintain an adequate blood flow to the brain during the operation a plastic tube may be inserted into the common and internal carotid arteries. It is removed when arterial closure is nearing completion.)

188. LIGATION OF THIRD PART OF SUBCLAVIAN ARTERY

i. An incision is made just above the clavicle, about 8 cm in length.

ii. The incision is deepened through the platysma to expose the external jugular vein and the deep fascia. The vein is ligated and divided.

iii. The deep fascia is divided to expose the omohyoid and its fascia and branches of the transverse cervical vessels.

iv. The omohyoid is mobilised to expose the subclavian artery. The upper and middle trunks of the brachial plexus lie above and laterally to the artery.

v. The artery is dissected free and ligated.

189. EXPOSURE OF INNOMINATE ARTERY

i. An incision is made along the right anterior margin of the sternomastoid and extended down over the manubrium sterni.

ii. The sternal head of the sternomastoid muscle is detached.

iii. The medial end of clavicle is exposed cleared and divided.

iv. The posterior aspect of the manubrium is cleared and the right portion of it divided with a Gigli saw. Elevation and retraction of the divided portion exposes the superior mediastinum.

v. In front of the innominate artery is the left innominate vein and the inferior thyroid veins. The latter veins are ligated and divided. To the right lies the right innominate vein and the superior vena cava. To the left lies the left common carotid artery. The vagus, recurrent laryngeal and phrenic nerves are well to the lateral side. Posteriorly lies the trachea and pleura.

vi. The artery is ligated. The aneurysm needle is passed from the lateral side.

vii. The sternum is replaced.

viii. The skin closed.

ix. An alternative exposure is obtained by dividing the skin and the manubrium sterni tranversely at the level of the second intercostal space.

190. EXPOSURE OF BRACHIAL ARTERY – MIDDLE PART

i. The limb is abducted, externally rotated and held in this position by placing the forearm on a table.

ii. An incision is made along the medial aspect of the biceps.

iii. The deep fascia is divided lateral to the basilic vein.

iv. The artery is dissected free of its veins and the median nerve which may be in front of it identified and preserved.

191. EXPOSURE OF TERMINAL PART OF BRACHIAL ARTERY

i. The forearm is supinated.

ii. An incision is made along the medial edge of the biceps tendon.

iii. The tendon and its muscle is mobilised and retracted laterally by dividing the deep fascia and the bicipital aponeurosis. The median basilic vein is drawn inwards.

iv. The artery is seen with the median nerve on its medial side.

192. EXPOSURE OF EXTERNAL ILIAC ARTERY
Extraperitoneal Approach

i. The inguinal hernia approach is employed with the incision extended laterally.

ii. Divide the external oblique, and mobilise the cord.

iii. Divide the internal oblique commencing at the internal ring and proceeding laterally, parallel with the inguinal ligament.

iv. Divide the fascia transversalis and preserve the inferior epigastric vessels.

v. The artery is displayed with the vein medial to it. Laterally the femoral and genitofemoral nerves are seen.

vi. The peritoneum is gently retracted upwards and the artery cleared for 2·5 cm. The aneurysm needle is passed from without inwards.

vii. From the point of view of collateral circulation in the leg this ligation is safer than femoral artery ligation.

193. EXPOSURE OF FEMORAL ARTERY UPPER TWO-THIRDS

i. An incision is made along a line drawn from the midinguinal point to the adductor tubercle.

ii. The incision is deepened to expose the sartorius, the long saphenous vein is preserved.

iii. The sartorius is mobilised laterally to expose the entire artery and vein.

iv. The fascial roof overlying the vessels is divided.

v. The saphenous nerve and the nerve to vastus medialis is preserved.

vi. The artery may be ligated at the base or apex of the femoral triangle or in the subsartorial canal. The profunda femoris usually arises 4 cm below the inguinal ligament, ligation below its origin aids the establishment of the collateral circulation.

194. EXPOSURES OF THE POPLITEAL ARTERY

With the patient supine the affected limb is moderately flexed at the hip and knee and externally rotated.

Exposure of the upper part of the popliteal artery

i. A longitudinal incision is made along the lower third of a line drawn from the midinguinal point to the adductor tubercle.

ii. The sartorius muscle is retracted backwards.

iii. The thin fascia immediately behind the tendinous distal end of the adductor magnus is divided and the underlying fat displaced posteriorly to expose the popliteal artery.

Exposure of the lower part of the popliteal artery

i. An incision is made parallel to and 1 cm behind the upper third of the medial border of the tibia.

ii. The deep fascia is incised in the line of the incision.

iii. The gastrocnemius muscle is retracted backwards and the popliteal neurovascular bundle exposed.

iv. The artery is dissected free from the vein which lies on its inner side.

v. The tendons of semitendinosus and gracilis are divided close to their insertions if necessary to increase the exposure.

(*Note:* To complete the exposure of the popliteal artery the medial head of the gastrocnemius and the sartorius and semimembranosus muscles are divided close to their bony attachments.)

195. EXPOSURE OF THE POSTERIOR TIBIAL AND PERONEAL ARTERIES (Henry)

i. A long incision is made 1 cm behind and parallel to the medial border of the tibia.

ii. The deep fascia is incised in the line of the incision.

iii. The fibrous origin of the soleus muscle from the middle third of the medial border of the tibia and the soleal line is divided.

iv. The soleus muscle is retracted backwards to expose the posterior tibial vessels and, further laterally, the peroneal vessels.

v. In the lower third of the leg the posterior tibial artery is covered only by deep fasciae.

196. FEMOROPOPLITEAL ARTERIAL BYPASS WITH REVERSED VEIN GRAFT

i. The patient is placed in the supine position with the affected lower limb slightly flexed at the hip and knee and externally rotated.

ii. An appropriate length of the ipsilateral long saphenous vein, with its tributaries ligated, is removed through one or more incisions. Any small holes demonstrated by flushing the graft through with saline are sutured. The proximal end is marked with a stitch.

iii. The common femoral artery is exposed.

iv. The upper or lower part of the popliteal artery is exposed using a medial approach.

v. Heparin is given intravenously.

vi. The proximal end of the vein graft is cut obliquely and anastomosed end-to-side to a segment of popliteal artery isolated between vascular clamps.

vii. The distal end of the graft is brought up to the groin through a subsartorial tunnel made with the finger or a tunneling instrument. Alternatively the graft may be placed subcutaneously in the saphenous vein bed.

viii. Excess graft is excised after extending the knee.

ix. The upper anastomosis to the common femoral artery is constructed.

x. Protamine sulphate is given to reverse the action of the heparin.

xi. The clamps are removed and the presence of pulsation well below the lower anastomosis is confirmed.

197. EXTRACTION OF AORTIC SADDLE EMBOLUS (Fogarty)

i. Intravenous heparin is given as soon as the diagnosis is made.

ii. Vertical incisions are made in the groins.

iii. The common femoral arteries are exposed and clamped immediately below the inguinal ligaments.

iv. A 1 cm longitudinal arteriotomy is made in one common femoral artery just above its bifurcation.

v. A Fogarty catheter is passed down through the superficial femoral to the ankle and as it is withdrawn the balloon is progressively inflated. This removes propagated clot. The superficial femoral artery is clamped to stop retrograde bleeding.

vi. The deep femoral artery is similarly cleared.

vii. The procedure is repeated on the opposite side.

viii. The clamp on either common femoral artery is removed, a Fogarty catheter is passed up into the aorta and part of the embolus is extracted with the distended balloon. A forceful gush of blood should follow and is controlled by the re-application of the clamp.

ix. The procedure is repeated on the opposite side to remove the remainder of the embolus.

x. The arteriotomies are carefully closed to avoid narrowing the vessels.

xi. The action of the heparin is reversed and the clamps are removed.

xii. The pulses are checked before wound closure.

(Note: i. Retrograde bleeding does not necessarily exclude the presence of distal clot.

ii. The Fogarty catheter may have to be passed several times before the arterial tree is completely clear.)

198. GRAFT REPLACEMENT OF ABDOMINAL AORTIC ANEURYSM

i. A long midline or paramedian incision is made.

ii. The peritoneal cavity is opened and the viscera and major arteries are examined.

iii. The small bowel is drawn out over the right wound edge and covered with moist packs. The transverse colon and greater omentum are drawn out over the top of the wound.

iv. The peritoneum over the aneurysm and common iliac arteries is divided, taking care to avoid damaging the ureters at the pelvic brim.

v. The third and fourth parts of the duodenum are mobilised and retracted to the right.

vi. The left renal vein crossing the neck of the aneurysm is identified and preserved.

vii. The neck of the aneurysm and the common iliac arteries are exposed with care to avoid damage to the iliac veins.

viii. The inferior mesenteric artery is divided between ligatures close to the aneurysm.

ix. The Dacron graft is pre-clotted.

x. Heparin is given intravenously.

xi. The aorta above the aneurysm and the common iliac arteries are clamped.

xi. The aneurysm is opened, thrombus is removed and retrograde bleeding from the lumbar arteries is stopped with transfixion sutures.

xii. The vessel ends are prepared for anastomosis by cutting along the junction between sac and vessel above and below.

xiii. The graft is sutured in above and below the sac.

xiv. Protamine sulphate is injected intravenously to reverse the action of the heparin.

xv. The distal clamps are removed.

xvi. The aortic clamp is replaced by compression of the artery between the finger and thumb and blood gradually permitted to flow through the graft.

xvii. The sac of the aneurysm is partially excised leaving enough to suture over the graft.

xviii. The posterior peritoneum is repaired.

xix. The viscera are returned to the abdominal cavity.

xx. The wound is closed.

199. MICROVASCULAR SURGERY – DIGITAL RE-IMPLANTATION

i. Special microsurgical instruments and a dissecting microscope giving a magnification of up to 25× are necessary. 10/0 sutures are used.

ii. A tourniquet is applied.

iii. The wounds are excised.

iv. The bone ends are aligned and immobilised.

v. At least one artery and two veins are anastomosed. Eight interrupted sutures are required to anastomose the 1 mm digital artery.

vi. The digital nerves are repaired, also under magnification.

vii. The tendons are repaired.

200. INFERIOR VENA CAVA LIGATION

i. The vessel may be approached through an upper paramedian incision (or extraperitoneally via an oblique or transverse abdominal incision).

ii. The peritoneal cavity is opened and the bowel packed off to expose the third part of the duodenum; it is mobilised to expose the inferior vena cava.

iii. The vessel is dissected circumferentially and the size of its lumen reduced to 1·5 cm by two encircling linen sutures or plastic clip.

Index

(Numbers refer to pages, not sections)